The Paperless Medical Office for Billers and Coders

SECOND EDITION

Using Harris CareTracker

Virginia Ferrari

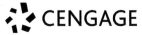

Australia • Brazil • Mexico • Singapore • United Kingdom • United States

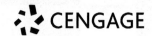

The Paperless Medical Office for Billers and Coders: Using Harris CareTracker,
2nd Edition

Virginia Ferrari

SVP, GM Skills & Global Product Management:
Jonathan Lau

Product Director: Matthew Seeley

Product Team Manager: Stephen Smith

Senior Director, Development:
Marah Bellegarde

Senior Content Development Manager:
Juliet Steiner

Content Developer: Kaitlin Schlicht

Product Assistant: Jessica Molesky

Marketing Manager: Jonathan Sheehan

Senior Content Project Manager:
Thomas Heffernan

Art Director: Angela Sheehan

Production Service: SPi Global

Cover Images: VAlex/Shutterstock.com,
Vectorphoto/Shutterstock.com, smartdesign91/
Shutterstock.com, Bryan Solomon/
Shutterstock.com, Blan-K/Shutterstock.com,
Aha-Soft/Shutterstock.com, RedKoala/
Shutterstock.com

For product information and technology assistance, contact us at
Cengage Customer & Sales Support, 1-800-354-9706.

For permission to use material from this text or product,
submit all requests online at **www.cengage.com/permissions**.
Further permissions questions can be emailed to
permissionrequest@cengage.com.

Library of Congress Control Number: 2017957038

ISBN: 978-1-337-61420-7

Cengage
20 Channel Street
Boston, MA 02210
USA

Cengage is a leading provider of customized learning solutions with employees residing in nearly 40 different countries and sales in more than 125 countries around the world. Find your local representative at: **www.cengage.com**.

Cengage products are represented in Canada by Nelson Education, Ltd.

For your course and learning solutions, visit **www.cengage.com**.

Purchase any of our products at your local college store or at our preferred online store **www.cengagebrain.com**.

Printed in the United States of America
Print Number: 02   Print Year: 2018

Contents

List of Activities

Preface

Electronic technology is the major means through which workers communicate in today's health care environment. *The Paperless Medical Office for Billers and Coders: Using Harris CareTracker, 2nd Edition* is an electronic health record solution that integrates instructional theory with state-of-the-art practice management and electronic medical record software.

Harris CareTracker PM and EMR is one of the most advanced cloud-based practice management systems (PM) and electronic medical records (EMR) in the industry. The product is certified through the Certification Commission for Health Information Technology (CCHIT®) and is used by thousands of providers throughout the country. The Harris CareTracker product provides state-of-the-art features and user-friendly software and is compliant with governmental mandates.

The PM side of Harris CareTracker is a sophisticated practice management system that automates time-consuming administrative tasks such as eligibility checks, scheduling, reminders, patient visit documentation, claims submission, and related billing and coding functions. Its features include:

- Interactive dashboards that prioritize work lists automatically
- A rules-based, front-end clinical editing tool that scrubs outgoing claims prior to submission
- An online code lookup software that boosts coding accuracy

The EMR side of Harris CareTracker monitors and measures all clinical data and prioritizes anything that needs attention. Some of the outstanding features of Harris CareTracker EMR include:

- Automatic refill requests
- Chart management
- Lab management
- Medication history
- Prescription (Rx) writing
- Report management

PURPOSE OF THE TEXT

The Paperless Medical Office for Billers and Coders: Using Harris CareTracker, 2nd Edition was written to fill a void in today's EHR training market and provide training specifically for financial functions and those PM and EMR activities that affect billing and coding. Many EHR training solutions are available but this workbook provides 8–10 hours of step-by-step training activities that simulate typical workflows in ambulatory health organizations related to the billing and coding functions. This workbook takes students through critical information on integrating EHR software into the medical practice, and then offers step-by-step guidance on how those principles can be applied using the Harris CareTracker PM and EMR software.

Chapters 1 and 2 include introductory activities in the Harris CareTracker PM and EMR software. Activities in Chapter 1 guide students through how to set up their computers for optimal performance, register their credentials, and create their personal Harris CareTracker training companies. Chapter 2 introduces the *Help* system and the purpose and location of key components of the EHR. Chapters 3 through 8 contain step-by-step front and back office functions related to billing and coding activities for students to complete. At the end of each activity, students will be asked to print a screenshot or report that captures the work they have completed. Students are encouraged to keep this documentation in an "assignments" folder, to submit to their instructor. Chapter 9 provides case studies without the benefit of step-by-step instructions. Completing the Chapter 9 case studies affirms proficiency using Harris CareTracker PM and EMR for billing and coding.

ORGANIZATION OF THE WORKBOOK

The Paperless Medical Office for Billers and Coders, 2nd Edition is organized to match the daily flow of an office. The first two chapters serve as an introduction to the Harris CareTracker PM and EMR software and how to navigate it. Beginning with Chapter 3, Patient Demographics and continuing throughout the workbook, students follow the logical sequence of what occurs from the time the patient registers and schedules an appointment through to processing the insurance claim form generated from the patient's visit and any related collection activities.

The following breakdown summarizes what is included in each chapter:

Chapter 1: Introduction to the Paperless Medical Office

This chapter discusses the core functions, advantages, and disadvantages of electronic health records. Students are introduced to administrative and clinical workflows in Harris CareTracker PM and EMR, and the online coding processes and EncoderPro.com. Students are also instructed on how to set up their computer for optimal functionality and create a Harris CareTracker training company.

Chapter 2: Introduction to Harris CareTracker PM and EMR

Students learn how to log in to Harris CareTracker in this chapter and use the *Help* system. Basic navigation functions of the *Main Menu, Home*, and *Dashboard* are presented here as well as the discussion of administrative features available within Harris CareTracker PM. Students will gain a firm understanding of using an electronic messaging system and will demonstrate their knowledge by performing messaging activities.

Chapter 3: Patient Demographics

In this chapter, students learn the fundamentals of entering patient demographics, registering new patients, and viewing and performing eligibility checks.

Chapter 4: Appointment Scheduling

Scheduling is the central theme of this chapter. Students will learn how to book appointments and how to check in patients, set operator preferences, create a batch, accept payments, print patient receipts, run a journal, and post the batch.

Chapter 5: Preliminary Duties in the EHR and Patient Work-Up

This chapter is where the EMR side of Harris CareTracker is introduced. Students will be introduced to the concept of Meaningful Use and receive training in how to activate the care management registries.

Students then learn the major applications of the *Clinical Today* module—the clinical or EMR side of Harris CareTracker. Because this workbook focuses on billing and coding, only minimal clinical-related activities will be performed. Student activities include viewing daily appointments, transferring patients, and tracking patients throughout the visit. In addition, students will learn how to retrieve the patient's EMR and update sections within the health history panes, update the patient care management application, and create and print a progress note.

Chapter 6: Completing the Visit

This chapter focuses on what occurs following the patient's examination. Students will learn how to complete the visit, resolve open encounters, and sign the progress note. In order to generate claims, charges must be captured for the patient's appointment. Students will enter procedure and diagnostic codes for billing purposes.

Chapter 7: Billing

Students switch back to administrative tasks in this chapter. Once the visit is completed, the billing activities begin. Creating a batch for billing activities, manually entering charges, and editing an unposted charge are just a few of the activities in this chapter. Users will also learn how to generate electronic and paper claims and perform activities related to electronic remittance.

Chapter 8: ClaimsManager and Collections

In this chapter, users will learn the functions of the *ClaimsManager* feature in Harris CareTracker and will check the status of unpaid or inactive claims. Students will learn how to generate patient statements, review collection status and transfer private pay balances, create custom collections letters, and navigate the collections process.

Chapter 9: Applied Learning for the Paperless Medical Office

This chapter is the finale of the workbook. It includes a comprehensive case study that tests users' knowledge and understanding of the material presented throughout the workbook without providing step-by-step instructions. Students build both competence and confidence from performing the activities in this chapter.

NEW TO THIS EDITION

The second edition of this text has been revised to provide greater student support. Updates include:

- A **Best Practices** guide at the beginning of the workbook outlines key tips for working in Harris Care-Tracker PM and EMR.
- A **Student Companion Website** includes some video tutorials and a mapping grid showing chapter activities you can reference for help when completing the Applied Learning Case Studies (Chapter 11).
- A **Critical Thinking** feature included throughout the chapters helps the students think about and address issues they may face on the job.
- **Required icons** appear next to chapter activities that are required in order to proceed. This helps prevent students from skipping over necessary activities.

As a result of these changes, activities in each chapter have been reorganized and some activities have also been rewritten for greater clarification. In addition to reorganizing the text and updating activities, some content updates have been made. Major content updates include:

- Focus on ICD-10 coding with reference to ICD-9 only for historical information
- Streamlined and clarified steps for building claims and processing remittance advice

FEATURES

The *Help* system within the Harris CareTracker software includes a plethora of educational materials and training tutorials that provide tips for using Harris CareTracker PM and EMR. In addition to text materials, the Harris CareTracker *Help* system provides training videos that walk users through each function within the system. Because this product is a live program, updated training materials containing the most recent information for Meaningful Use, ICD-10, and HIPAA are available.

The 8–10 hours of hands-on, step-by-step training activities include Professionalism Connections and Critical Thinking components. Students will learn how to use the different functions of the Harris CareTracker software to meet billing and coding needs critical to the financial health of the practice.

- Unique features of the text also include: **Learning Objectives** state chapter goals and outcomes.
- The **Real-World Connection** feature at the start of each chapter contains information regarding a day in the life of a medical assistant working in a medical practice using electronic health records. The "real world" scenarios are meant to stimulate thought and critical thinking.
- The **Professionalism Connection** boxes provide helpful information on how students can best present themselves in a professional manner. This includes showing proficiency in assigned tasks as well as communicating and interacting effectively with patients and staff.
- **Spotlight** boxes highlight important material included throughout the text. It is critical that users of EHR software are familiar with this information.

- **Alert** boxes present critical information to know when completing activities in Harris CareTracker PM and EMR.
- **Required icons** alert students to activities that are required within a chapter in order for them to proceed with that chapter and later activities.
- **Tip** boxes provide helpful hints for using Harris CareTracker PM and EMR.
- **FYI** boxes provide details on functions of Harris CareTracker PM and EMR that are available in real-world settings but are not available in your student version of Harris CareTracker.
- **Critical Thinking** boxes help students think about and address issues they may face on the job.
- The Step-by-Step **Activities** give instructions on how to complete front and back office functions in Harris CareTracker PM and EMR. They feature detailed information on steps to be performed as well as screenshots that illustrate key steps.
- The **Case Studies** provide additional opportunity for students to test their ability to complete key chapter activities without the benefit of step-by-step instructions.

DISCLAIMER

Due to the evolving nature and continuous upgrades of real-world EMRs such as this one, as you log in and work in your student version of Harris CareTracker, there may be a slightly different look to your live screen from the screenshots provided in the workbook.

Keep in mind that you will be asked to work in "current dates" when completing activities, so your appointment and encounter dates will not match those used in the workbook screenshots.

When prompted, follow the instructions given in the workbook to complete the activities.

LEARNING PACKAGE FOR THE STUDENT
Student Companion Website

Cengage's Student Companion Website to accompany *The Paperless Medical Office: Using Harris CareTracker, 2nd Edition* is a complementary resource that includes additional support such as a blank Patient Registration Form for additional practice, some video tutorials, and a mapping grid showing which chapter activities you can reference for help when completing the Applied Learning Case Studies (Chapter 9). To access the Student Companion Website from CengageBrain, go to http://www.cengagebrain.com, and key ISBN 9781337614191 in the **Search** window. Locate the *The Paperless Medical Office: Using Harris CareTracker, 2nd Edition* and click on the title. Scroll to the bottom of the page and click on the **Free Materials** tab, then **Save to MyHome**. Once you have added it to "My Home," click on the product under "My Products" for access to the Student Companion Website.

TEACHING PACKAGE FOR THE INSTRUCTOR
Instructor Companion Website

(ISBN 978-1-337-61422-1)

Spend less time planning and more time teaching with Cengage's Instructor Companion Website to accompany *The Paperless Medical Office: Using Harris CareTracker, 2nd Edition*. As an instructor, you will have access to all of your resources online, anywhere and at any time. All instructor resources can be accessed by going to www.cengage .com/login to create a unique user log-in. The password protected instructor resources include the following:

- Answer keys for activities and case studies.
- Mapping of the Applied Learning Case Studies (Chapter 9) to the in-text Activity number for reference.
- Spreadsheet showing which patients appear in which activities as well as what activities are required.

ABOUT THE AUTHOR

Virginia Ferrari is a former adjunct faculty member at Solano Community College in the Career Technical Education/Business division, where she taught medical front office, medical coding, and small business courses. In addition, she has been a contributing author for other Cengage Learning textbooks, including the Seventh and Eighth Editions of *Medical Assisting: Administrative and Clinical Competencies* and the Second Edition of *Clinical Medical Assisting: A Professional, Field Smart Approach to the Workplace*. Prior to joining Solano Community College, Virginia served as the manager of extended services for one of the fastest-growing physician networks in the San Francisco Bay area. In addition to overseeing the conversion and implementation of electronic medical records, she served on the Best Practice Committee, Customer Satisfaction Committee, Pilot Project for Risk Adjust Coding, and Team Up for Health, a national collaborative for Diabetes Self-Management Education. Virginia holds dual bachelor degrees in sociology and family and consumer studies from Central Washington University and a master's degree in health administration from the University of Phoenix. Virginia also holds certification from the National Healthcareer Association as a Certified Electronic Health Record Specialist (CEHRS). Virginia is a previous member of the AAMA Editorial Advisory Committee, and a current member of the AAMA Leadership Committee.

System Requirements for Harris CareTracker

MINIMUM REQUIREMENTS

- Intel core or Xeon processor
- Operating System: Windows 7, Windows 8, Windows 10, iPad IOS6
- Windows 7: 8 GB
- Microsoft Internet Explorer 11
- Acrobat Reader
- Adobe Flash
- Java
- 1024 × 768 resolution

THIRD-PARTY SOFTWARE

Third-party software (such as Yahoo! and Google toolbars, or Norton and McAfee, etc.) does not follow the rules setup in Internet options; therefore, it tends to block Harris CareTracker functionality with respect to pop-ups. If this does happen, then you need to add training.caretracker.com and rapidrelease.caretracker.com to the allowed or safe sites lists of those programs. Follow the instructions in the next section, Internet Settings Add as Trusted Site.

INTERNET SETTINGS

Add as Trusted Site

1. Open Internet Explorer browser window.
2. On the menu bar, click Tools and then select Internet Options from the menu. Internet Explorer displays the Internet Options dialog box.
3. Click the Security tab and then click Trusted Sites.
4. Click Sites. Internet Explorer displays the Trusted Sites dialog box.
5. In the Add this website to the zone box, type: training.caretracker.com.
6. Click Add. Internet Explorer adds the address to trusted sites.
7. Repeat steps 5 and 6 for rapidrelease.caretracker.com.
8. Deselect the Require server verification (https:) for all sites in this zone checkbox.
9. Click Close to close the Trusted Sites box.
10. Click OK on the Internet Options box to save your changes.

Compatibility View Settings

1. In Internet Explorer 11, launch the website for which you want to disable Compatibility View (www .cengage.com/caretracker).
2. If the menu bar is not visible, press the **Alt** key to display the browser menu.
3. On the browser menu, click the Tools > Compatibility View Settings. The browser opens the Compatibility View Settings window.
4. In the "Websites you've added to Compatibility View" section, remove caretracker.com if it appears there.

BANDWIDTH RECOMMENDATIONS

If there are multiple workstations utilizing Harris CareTracker, then each will require a minimum of 300kb of bandwidth per active workstation with a DSL or Cable connection. For a T1 or Dedicated connection, a minimum of 60kb per workstation is required.

RECOMMENDED SCREEN RESOLUTION

The recommended screen resolution is 1024 $\times$ 768.

SUPPORTED BROWSER

Harris CareTracker supports only Internet Explorer 11 for desktop devices. Safari for iPad may also be used. Mozilla Firefox and Google Chrome are not yet supported.

Best Practices for Harris CareTracker

Certain best practices should be followed whenever you are working in Harris CareTracker. A list of these best practices is provided below. Continue reading for more information on these best practices.

- Before beginning work each day, check the News application in CareTracker for updates from Harris CareTracker and Cengage. To do so, click on the Home Module and then click on the News tab.
- When you need to complete an activity, read all of the activity directions first, before completing any steps.
- Check your browser. Use only Internet Explorer 11 (IE 11) or Safari for iPad.
- Check Compatibility View settings. "Display intranet sites in Compatibility View" and "Use Microsoft compatibility lists" should be unchecked.
- Clear your cache each time you start working in Harris CareTracker.
- If you receive a "Duplicate Session" error message, close your browser window. Then open a new Internet Explorer browser window. In the new window, select File > New Session.
- When directed to "print," if a print button is not available in Harris CareTracker, take a screenshot of your work.
- Properly log out when you are finished working.
- For technical support questions, check your student companion website for solutions. If you can't find a solution to your issue, contact Cengage.

Check Your Browser

Harris CareTracker supports only Internet Explorer 11 and Safari for iPad.

To Determine Your Browser

You can determine the basic type of browser you are using by looking at the icon at the bottom of your computer screen, in the Start Menu, on the Desktop, or on your Task Bar. Internet Explorer or Safari for iPad are required for using Harris CareTracker. **Figure 1** shows the Internet Explorer icon. **Figure 2** shows the Safari icon

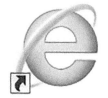

Figure 1
Internet Explorer
Icon

Used with permission from Microsoft

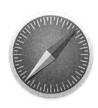

Figure 2
Safari Icon

Used with permission of Apple Inc.

(which is compatible with Harris CareTracker for iPads only). **Figure 3** shows other icons that are *not* compatible with Harris CareTracker (Google Chrome, Microsoft Edge, and Mozilla Firefox).

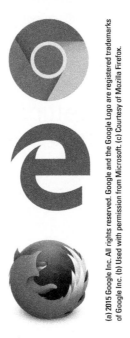

(a) 2015 Google Inc. All rights reserved. Google and the Google Logo are registered trademarks of Google Inc. (b) Used with permission from Microsoft. (c) Courtesy of Mozilla Firefox.

Figure 3 Google Chrome, Microsoft Edge, and Mozilla Firefox Icons

To Determine Your Browser Version

There are multiple versions of Internet Explorer. You must be working in Internet Explorer 11 to use Harris CareTracker. To determine which version you have, click on the Internet Explorer icon on your device. In the browser window, click on "Help" to bring up the Help menu (**Figure 4**). Click "About Internet Explorer", and you will see the pop up showing what version of IE you are using (**Figure 5**).

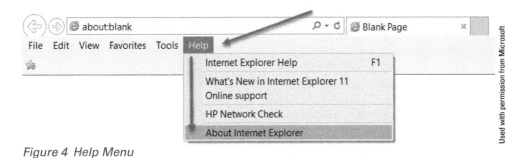

Used with permission from Microsoft

Figure 4 Help Menu

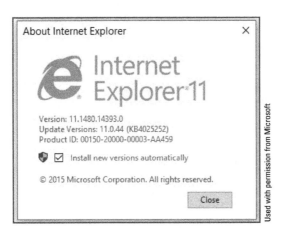

Used with permission from Microsoft

Figure 5 About Internet Explorer

To Locate Internet Explorer in Windows 10

Newer Windows computers may not have Internet Explorer installed and you will need to install prior to working in Harris CareTracker. To locate IE 11 in Windows 10, select the Start button and search for "Internet Explorer." If IE 11 is installed, you will see it pop up at the top of the search results. Search Microsoft's Support page for more help if needed, or to install IE 11 on your Windows computer.

Check Compatibility View Settings

You will need to change your Compatibility View Settings as follows.

1. Open up Internet Explorer 11 (IE 11).
2. Click on the Tools menu tab.
3. Select the Compatibility View settings option (**Figure 6**).

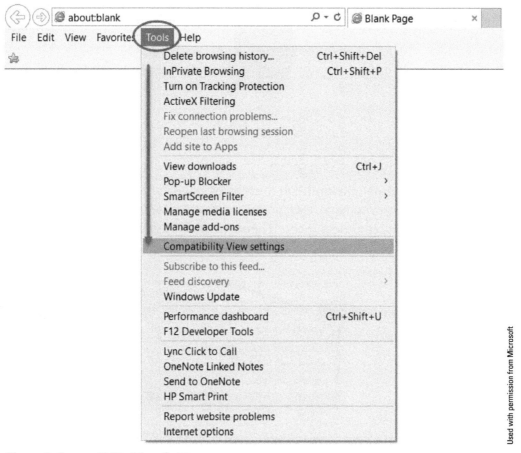

Figure 6 Compatibility View Settings

4. In the resulting pop-up, uncheck the "Display intranet sites in Compatibility View" option (**Figure 7**).
5. Uncheck "Use Microsoft compatibility lists" (Figure 7).
6. Click Close.

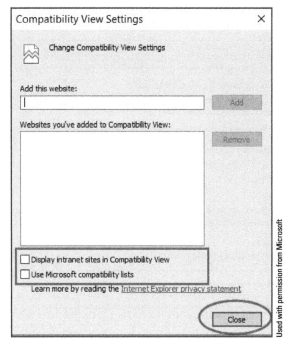

Figure 7 Change Compatibility View Settings

Clear Your Cache

You should clear your cache each time you begin working in CareTracker. To clear your cache in Internet Explorer 11:

1. Open an Internet Explorer® browser window.
2. From the *Tools* menu, select *Internet Options*. Windows® displays the *Internet Options* dialog box.
3. On the *General* tab, in the *Browsing history* section, click *Delete...* (**Figure 8**). Windows® displays the *Delete Browsing History* dialog box.

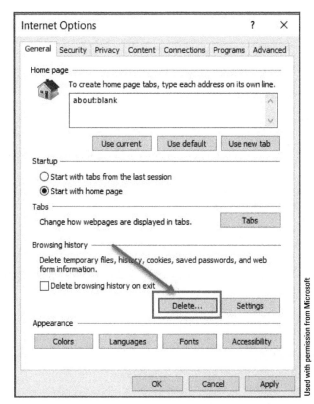

Figure 8 Delete Browsing History

4. Deselect the *Preserve Favorites website data* checkbox (**Figure 9**).

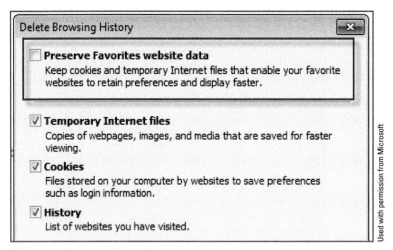

Figure 9 Preserve Favorites

5. Select the *Temporary Internet files and website files, Cookies and website data,* and *History* checkboxes only.
6. Click *Delete*.
7. Click *OK* when finished.

To clear your cache in Safari for iPad:

1. Tap *Settings* from your iPad® home screen.
2. Tap *Safari*® from the *Settings* pane on the left. The *Safari*® *Pane* displays *Clear History, Clear Cache,* and *Clear Cookies* at the bottom (**Figure 10**).

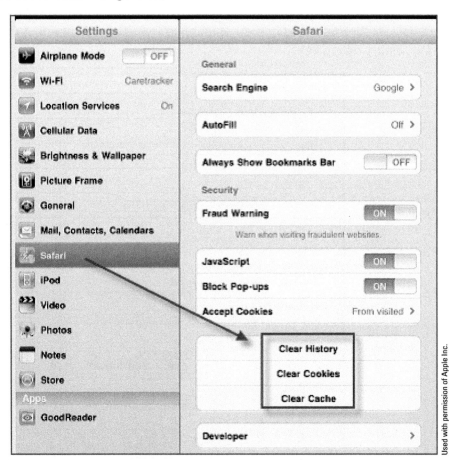

Figure 10 Safari Clear Cache

3. Tap *Clear History*. iPad® displays a confirmation window.
4. Tap *Clear* in the confirmation window.
5. Repeat steps 3 and 4 to clear your cache and cookies (refer to Figure 10).

Resolve a "Duplicate Session" Error Message

If you receive a "Duplicate Session" error message, close your browser window. Open a new Internet Explorer browser window. In the new window, select File > New Session. You should now be able to access Harris CareTracker.

Take a Screenshot

Throughout the text you will be instructed to "print" or in some cases, take a screenshot, of your work to submit to your instructor as confirmation of activity completion. To take a screenshot with your PC:

1. Find the screen you need to print out (this will usually be noted in your "end of activity print instruction").
2. Using your keyboard commands, take a screenshot. Depending on the computer you are using, the way you take a screenshot may vary. Typically, a screenshot can be captured using the Print Screen [PrtSc] key on your computer. Some users may need to press the key [Alt] and [PrtSc] to capture only the active window.
3. Open a Word document.
4. Using the Paste command, paste the image from the screen onto your Word document. This can also be accomplished by either right-clicking your mouse and choosing one of the Paste options, or by left-clicking anywhere in the Word document and pressing the keys [Ctrl] and [V] to paste the image onto the Word document.
5. Save the Word document and submit the document to your instructor as advised (electronically or paper).

Log Out of Harris CareTracker

It is important to properly log out of CareTracker when you are done with your session. Do not simply close the window, but instead, click on *Log Off* in Harris CareTracker (**Figure 11**).

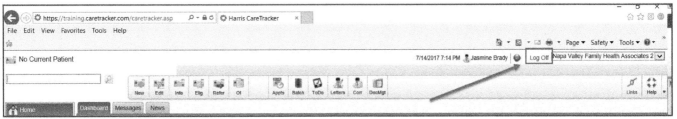

Figure 11 Properly Log Off Harris CareTracker PM and Physician EMR

Courtesy of Harris CareTracker PM and Physician EMR

Contact Cengage for Technical Support When Needed

If you have technical support questions while working through the activities in *The Paperless Medical Office*, check your student companion website for help. You can access your student companion website through logging in or creating a free student account at login.cengage.com, clicking on Find Free Study Tools, searching for and adding the ISBN 9781337614191, and then clicking on the product under My Products. If you are unable to resolve your issue through the support posted to the student companion website, then contact Cengage technical support at www.cengage.com/support.

 ALERT! WARNING!! Do not purchase a "used textbook", as the credentials would have already been registered and cannot be used again. You must have a new textbook with your own credentials in order to be able to create your training company for work in Harris CareTracker.

Introduction to the Paperless Medical Office

Learning Objectives

1. Describe core functions, advantages, and disadvantages of electronic health records.
2. Describe administrative and clinical workflows in Harris CareTracker PM and EMR.
3. Introduction to online coding processes and ClaimsManager the claims software in Harris CareTracker PM and EMR.
4. Set up your computer for optimal functionality when using Harris CareTracker PM and EMR.
5. Create a Harris CareTracker training company.

Real-World Connection

Welcome to Napa Valley Family Health Associates (NVFHA), your Harris CareTracker training company! Our practice is located in the beautiful Napa Valley in California. The practice consists of four providers, six medical assistants, one X-ray technician, and a medical lab scientist who oversees our laboratory. As a medical assisting student, you will rotate among our four providers:

- Amir Raman, DO (Specialty—Internal Medicine)
- Anthony Brockton, MD (Specialty—Family Practice)
- Rebecca Ayerick, MD (Specialty—Family Practice/Pediatrics)
- Gabrielle Torres, NP (Specialty—Family Practice)

We are a busy family health center and take care of patients across the lifespan. To be considered for a job in our practice, you must have a caring attitude, have strong administrative and clinical skills, and get along well with people of all ages and all socioeconomic backgrounds.

We are a practice that believes in a proactive approach to health care. We look for ways to improve patient outcomes while driving down health care costs. As a matter of fact, we recently applied for and received NCQA Patient-Centered Medical Home (PCMH) Recognition. The PCMH is a care delivery model whereby patient treatment is coordinated through their primary care provider to ensure the patient receives the necessary care when and where they need it, in a manner they can understand. Becoming a PCMH is a way of organizing primary care that emphasizes care coordination and communication to transform primary care into "what patients want it to be." Medical homes can lead to higher quality and lower costs and can improve patients' and providers' experience of care. We chose Harris CareTracker PM and EMR as our electronic health record system because of its robust functions and reporting capabilities, which are essential to a PCMH model.

This workbook focuses on technical skills, but do not be surprised if you learn a few other skills along the way! Throughout the text, you will be challenged to think critically and perform to the best of your ability. Your first challenge is to carefully read the instructions and implement all of the settings for the activities/features outlined in this first chapter. Failure to implement the recommended settings may result in an inability to perform some activities. Let's get started!

CORE FUNCTIONS OF THE EMR/EHR

Learning Objective 1: Describe core functions, advantages, and disadvantages of electronic health records.

The electronic record has many features designed to improve patient care and staff efficiency. The type of software that a medical practice selects will depend on many factors, including the type of practice, the goals of the practice, the cost of the software, and the individual preferences of the clinicians and staff.

Advantages of Electronic Medical/Health Records

An EMR system is an electronic platform that facilitates the needs of a medical practice. An advantage of using a fully integrated practice management and EMR such as Harris CareTracker is that it automates the overall workflow to the greatest extent possible to achieve the maximum amount of practice efficiency. Patient care coordination is improved, and there is a demonstrated reduction in errors, which previously resulted from illegible notes or prescriptions.

Disadvantages of the Electronic Health Record

EHRs have many benefits, but there are also a few pitfalls. In an article by the National Center for Biotechnology Information (Menachemi & Collum, 2011), it was noted that despite the growing consensus on benefits of EHR functionalities, there are some potential disadvantages associated with this technology. These include financial issues, changes in workflow, temporary loss of productivity associated with EHR adoption, privacy and security concerns, problems that occur when the system goes down, and other unintended consequences.

Recently, patients and providers have begun expressing concern over privacy issues related to EHRs and the personal information collected by the federal government. The Affordable Care Act (ACA) mandates the Internal Revenue Service (IRS) as the collection and enforcement arm for the federal government, which troubles many Americans. In addition, as the Department of Health and Human Services (HHS) issues additional rules pertaining to the ACA, there is more intrusion into a patient's medical files, and the patient's privacy is being sacrificed.

The possible repeal and replacement of the ACA is an ongoing debate in Congress, and may result in slight or significant changes to the law. Absent any changes in the law, it is expected that some of the rules and regulations will be changed to fix some shortcomings and deficiencies.

ADMINISTRATIVE AND CLINICAL WORKFLOWS IN HARRIS CARETRACKER

Learning Objective 2: Describe administrative and clinical workflows in Harris CareTracker PM and EMR.

Workflow is defined as how tasks are performed throughout the office (usually in a specific order), for example, the patient is checked in, insurance cards are scanned, copay is collected, the patient is taken to the exam room where vital signs are taken/recorded, and so on (**Figure 1-1**).

Practice management (PM) software runs the business side of health care, from registering a new patient and scheduling patient visits to coding and billing the patient encounter and generating monthly reports. Harris CareTracker PM software can be customized to user preferences. PM software maximizes provider productivity and meets rigorous scheduling demands. Alert messages, a master index, and insurance profiles help reduce error and administrative expenses during registration and charge entry.

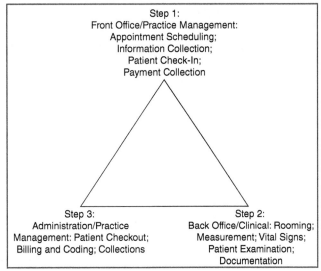

FIGURE 1-1   Patient Flow

The EMR side of Harris CareTracker focuses on the clinical side, encompassing documentation in the patient's medical record and how use of a certified EMR supports Meaningful Use as defined by the federal government, which sets incentive payments to providers for using an EHR and penalties for not using an EHR.

CODING FUNDAMENTALS

Learning Objective 3: Introduction to online coding processes and ClaimsManager, the claims software in Harris CareTracker PM and EMR.

Most EHRs have features that automate the coding process. Although the features of each EHR may vary, the codes are checked for accuracy by a coding specialist or program. Harris CareTracker's automated coding process is the *ClaimsManager* feature, which utilizes *EncoderPro.com*. *EncoderPro.com* is Harris CareTracker's partner for online code verification, which can be run to verify that all procedure, diagnosis, and modifier codes entered for a patient are correct.

To receive reimbursement, every service submitted for payment must be documented in the patient's medical record. The integration of automated coding with the billing system facilitates claims processing.

This billing and coding workbook focuses on medical assistants tasked with responsibilities for collections and the revenue cycle and familiarizes them with coding and compliance, claims scrubber programs, and why it is important for billers and coders to be familiar with and be proficient in using EHRs. Billers and coders will need to be familiar with ICD-10 diagnosis coding, the code set that replaced ICD-9 codes and is effective from October 1, 2015. Medical coders and billers must be up to date on the latest information related to coding, chart auditing, and insurance reimbursement. You must demonstrate familiarity and accuracy of ICD, CPT®, and HCPCS coding and comply with HIPAA standards for billing and insurance.

SET UP COMPUTER FOR OPTIMAL FUNCTIONALITY

Learning Objective 4: Set up your computer for optimal functionality when using Harris CareTracker PM and EMR.

In order to complete activities in Harris CareTracker, you must first set up your computer for optimal functionality. You will then register your credentials and create your Harris CareTracker training company. Because it may take up to 24 hours for your student company to be created, you will complete these activities now.

Readiness Requirements

In order to use Harris CareTracker, you must meet the minimum system requirements and update your browser settings. You'll walk through these requirements in the activities in this chapter. In addition, the most current System Requirements can be found on your student companion site.

 TIP You will find up-to-date *System Requirements and Recommendations* in the *Help* system of Harris CareTracker at *Help > Contents tab > System Requirements & Recommendations folder.* Chapter 2 will introduce you to *Help* and the various content and training available.

To use Harris CareTracker PM and EMR, your computer must have Internet Explorer® version 11. Other browsing software (outside of Safari® for iPad®) may work differently with the application. See the System Requirements section for further technology requirements. Chrome and Firefox are not currently supported. While iPads are compatible with Harris CareTracker, Macs cannot be used to register an access code, also known as your credentials. In an EHR, credentials are the login information required to access the software, which is the assigned username and password.

Disable Third-Party Toolbars

Remove all third-party toolbars (Google, Yahoo!, Bing, AOL, etc.) from Internet Explorer®. Third-party toolbars cause random performance and functionality issues within Harris CareTracker PM and EMR. Complete Activity 1-1 to disable toolbars.

 ## Activity 1-1
Disable Toolbars

1. Open an Internet Explorer® browser window.

2. Right-click on the menu bar. The browser displays a list of toolbars. Active toolbars appear with a check mark to the left of the name (Figure 1-2).

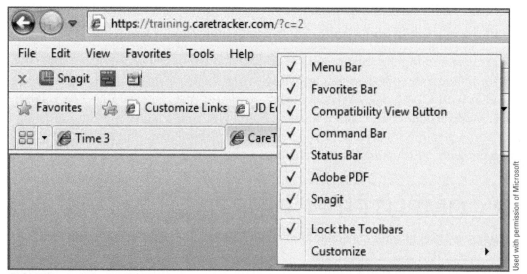

FIGURE 1-2 Disable Toolbars

3. Uncheck the toolbars you want to disable (Google, Yahoo!, Bing, AOL, etc. if displaying). Internet Explorer® disables the toolbar if that toolbar does not have a check mark next to it.

Setting Up Tabbed Browsing

Tabbed browsing allows you to open multiple websites in a single browser window. It is very important to set this up to access several patient charts at one time in a single browser. This will make switching between patients much easier and enables you to have multiple items open on the task bar. Complete Activity 1-2 to set up tabbed browsing.

 ### Activity 1-2
Set Up Tabbed Browsing

1. Open an Internet Explorer® browser window.

2. Select *Tools > Internet Options* from the browser menu. The *Internet Options* dialog box displays.

3. In the *Tabs* section, click *Tabs*. The *Tabbed Browsing Settings* dialog box displays.

4. Select the following options noted below and in Figure 1-3:

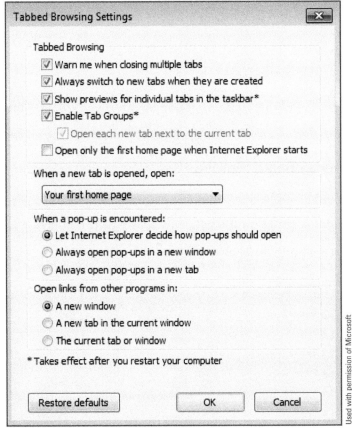

FIGURE 1-3   Tabbed Browsing Settings

- Warn me when closing multiple tabs
- Always switch to new tabs when they are created
- Show previews for individual tabs in the taskbar*
- Enable Tab Groups*
- When a new tab is opened, open: Your first home page

- When a pop-up is encountered: Let Internet Explorer decide on how pop-ups should open
- Open links from other programs in: A new window

Takes effect after you restart your computer

5. Click *OK* to close the *Tabbed Browsing Settings* box.

6. Click *OK* on the *Internet Options* box to save your changes.

Disable Pop-Up Blocker

A pop-up window is a small web browser window that appears on top of the website you are viewing. This allows you to avoid having to navigate away from the current window you are viewing. Harris CareTracker PM and EMR uses the pop-up mechanism, enabling an efficient workflow. Many computers have firewall protectors that alleviate nonsense pop-up ads from displaying as you work on a website. However, you must enable pop-ups to use the functionality within Harris CareTracker PM and EMR. Complete Activity 1-3 to turn off pop-up blocker in Internet Explorer® and Safari®.

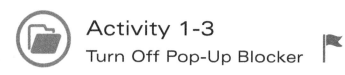

Activity 1-3
Turn Off Pop-Up Blocker

1. To disable pop-up blocker in Internet Explorer, open an Internet Explorer® browser window.

2. Select *Tools > Pop-up Blocker > Turn Off Pop-up Blocker* from the browser menu.

To disable pop-up blocker in Safari® for iPad®:

1. Tap *Settings* from your iPad® home screen.

2. Tap *Safari®* from the *Settings* panes on the left. The *Safari® Pane* displays the browser options.

3. Tap *Block Pop-ups* to turn off pop-up blocker (Figure 1-4).

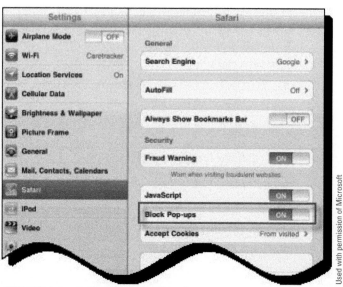

FIGURE 1-4   Safari® Pop-Up Blocker

Change the Page Setup

It is important to change the default margin, header, and footer settings to print letters, forms, and claims in Harris CareTracker PM and EMR. Complete Activity 1-4 to change page setup.

Activity 1-4
Change Page Setup

1. Open an Internet Explorer® browser window (one such as your Harris CareTracker training company). **Note**: You must have an actual website up, not just a blank/new tab.

2. On the browser menu bar, click *File*. Then choose *Page Setup* from the menu. Internet Explorer® launches the *Page Setup* dialog box.

3. Delete the values in the *Margins* (*inches*) fields. Leaving these fields blank will automatically set their value to zero.

4. Select *Empty* in each of the *Header* and *Footer* fields. Click *OK*.

Downloading Plug-Ins

A plug-in is a program that works with Harris CareTracker PM and EMR to give added functionality. Follow each link to download the required plug-in for free, if you don't have the plug-in already.

- Adobe Reader (*www.adobe.com, search for "Reader"*)
  - *To view, navigate, and print PDF files.*
- Adobe Flash (*www.adobe.com, search for "Flash Player"*)
  - *To view animation and interactive content.*
- Java (*www.java.com*)
  - *To run applications and applets that use Java technology. Java is required to view prerecorded sessions.*

Adding Trusted Sites

Add *training.caretracker.com* and *rapidrelease.caretracker.com* to the trusted site list. Otherwise some functionality may be blocked, such as running ActiveX controls and installing browser plug-ins. Adding trusted sites also allows your computer to distinguish between secured sites and harmful sites. Complete Activity 1-5 to add trusted sites.

Activity 1-5
Add Harris CareTracker to Trusted Sites

1. Open an Internet Explorer® browser window.

2. On the menu bar, click *Tools* and then select *Internet Options* from the menu. Internet Explorer® displays the *Internet Options* dialog box.

3. Click the *Security* tab and then click *Trusted sites*.

4. Click *Sites*. Internet Explorer® displays the *Trusted sites* dialog box.

5. Deselect the *Require server verification (https:) for all sites in this zone* checkbox.

6. In the *Add this website to the zone* box, type: training.caretracker.com.

7. Click *Add*. Internet Explorer® adds the address to trusted sites.

8. In the *Add this website to the zone* box, type: *rapidrelease.caretracker.com*.

9. Click *Add*. Internet Explorer® adds the address to trusted sites (Figure 1-5).

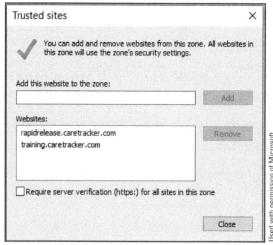

FIGURE 1-5 *Trusted Sites*

10. Click *Close* to close the *Trusted sites* box.

11. Click *OK* on the *Internet Options* box to save your changes.

Clearing the Cache

The cache is a space in your computer's hard drive and random access memory (RAM) where your browser saves copies of recently visited web pages. Typically, these items are stored in the *Temporary Internet Files* folder. It is important to clear your cache on a regular basis and at every release for Harris CareTracker PM and EMR to function more efficiently.

TIP Important!! You must first clear your cache each time you log in to Harris CareTracker PM and EMR. If you are already logged in, log out of Harris CareTracker PM and EMR before clearing your cache.

Activity 1-6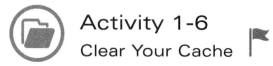
Clear Your Cache

To clear cache in Internet Explorer® 11:

1. Open an Internet Explorer® browser window.

2. From the Internet Explorer® *Tools* menu, select *Internet Options*. Windows® displays the *Internet Options* dialog box.

3. On the *General* tab, in the *Browsing history* section, click *Delete*. Windows® displays the *Delete Browsing History* dialog box.

4. Deselect the *Preserve Favorites website data* checkbox.

5. Select the *Temporary Internet files and website files, Cookies and website data,* and *History* checkboxes only.

6. Click *Delete.*

7. Click *OK* when finished.

To clear cache in Safari® for iPad®:

1. Tap *Settings* from your iPad® home screen.

2. Tap *Safari*® from the *Settings* panes on the left. The *Safari*® *Pane* displays the *Clear History, Clear Cookies,* and *Clear Cache* at the bottom (Figure 1-6).

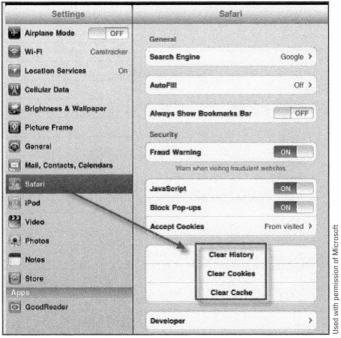

FIGURE 1-6   *Safari*® *Clear Settings*

3. Tap *Clear History.* iPad® displays a confirmation window.

4. Tap *Clear* in the confirmation window.

5. Repeat steps 3 and 4 to clear your cache and cookies (refer to Figure 1-6).

Setting Your Home Page

Your home page is displayed when Internet Explorer® first opens. You can choose to set Harris CareTracker PM and EMR as your home page if necessary.

Activity 1-7
Setting Harris CareTracker as Home Page

1. Open an Internet Explorer® browser window.

2. Select *Tools > Internet Options* from the browser menu. The *Internet Options* dialog box displays.

3. In the *Address* box of the *Home page* section, type: *https://www.cengage.com/CareTracker* (Figure 1-7).

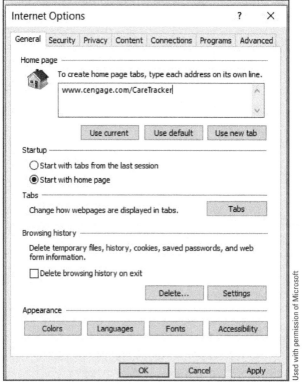

FIGURE 1-7   Home Page

4. Click *OK*. Harris CareTracker PM and EMR will display as your home page the next time you open Internet Explorer®.

Disable Download Blocking

Complete Activity 1-8 to disable download blocking.

 ## Activity 1-8
Disable Download Blocking

1. Open an Internet Explorer® browser window.

2. Select *Tools > Internet Options* from the browser menu. The browser displays the *Internet Options* dialog box.

3. Click the *Security* tab.

4. If not already defaulted to *Internet*, click the *Internet* (globe) link.

5. Click the *Custom level...* button.

6. Scroll down to the *Downloads* section.

7. In the *File Download* section, click *Enable*. Click *OK*.

8. Click *OK* in the *Internet Options* window to close it.

Now that you have set your computer to the required settings to work in Harris CareTracker PM and EMR, you will register your credentials and log in to begin your training.

REGISTER YOUR CREDENTIALS AND CREATE YOUR HARRIS CARETRACKER TRAINING COMPANY

Learning Objective 5: Create a Harris CareTracker training company.

You will be assigned a user name and password (your credentials) to log in to Harris CareTracker PM and EMR. Your preassigned user name and password can be found on the inside front cover of this workbook. Your password must be changed the first time you log in to Harris CareTracker PM and EMR. You will also be prompted to change your password every 90 days for security reasons. The password must consist of at least eight characters with one capital letter and one numeric character. As best practice, write your new password and the date created on the inside cover of your textbook each time you change it.

Before beginning any activities, clear your cache as instructed in Activity 1-6 for Internet Explorer or for iPad. If you are using a personal computer (PC), only work in Internet Explorer®. Use Safari® for iPad®. Once the cache has been cleared, you may continue by registering your credentials and creating your Harris CareTracker training company (Activity 1-9).

Activity 1-9

Register Your Credentials and Create Your Harris CareTracker PM and EMR Training Company

1. Go to *http://www.cengage.com/CareTracker* (Figure 1-8).

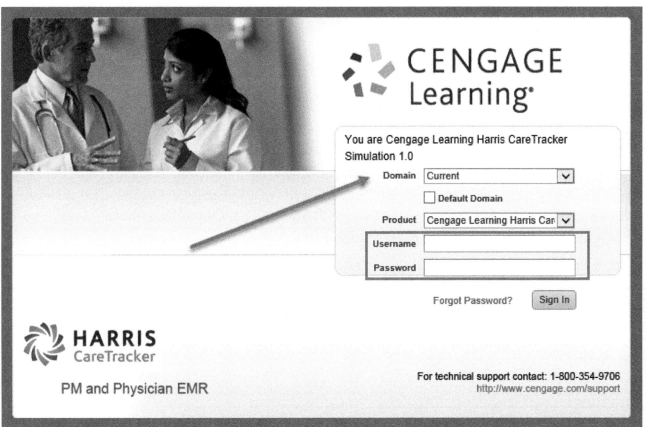

FIGURE 1-8   Login Screen

2. The "Domain" is set to *Current*. Do not change this setting—leave as is.

3. The *Product* list is set to "Cengage Learning Harris CareTracker Simulation 1.0" by default. Leave as is.

4. In the *Username* box, enter the username preassigned to you on the inside front cover of this workbook.

5. In the *Password* box, enter your password. If this is your first time logging in to Harris CareTracker PM and EMR, use the preassigned password located on the inside front cover of this workbook. On your first login, you will be prompted to change your temporary password and complete the *Security Information* and *General Information* fields in the *Operators Settings* dialog box.

TIP Both the username and password are case sensitive.
Your new password:

- Must differ from your old password by at least one character

- Must consist of at least eight characters

- Must contain at least one capital letter and one number; for example: Password5

- Must be reentered in the *Verify Password* field

---

6. Complete the *Security Information* fields by selecting a security question and providing the answer.

7. In the *General Information* fields, enter your *Phone* number (best contact), your *Email* (best contact), and skip the *Direct Email Address* field.

8. Record your new password on the inside cover of this workbook and the date the password was created. This allows for easy reference in case of a lost or expired password.

9. After changing your password and completing the *Security* and *General* information fields, click *Save*. A message will display indicating that your operator settings have been updated.

10. Close out of the *Success* box. Harris CareTracker will now create your training account and you will receive a notification email when the process is complete. Figure 1-9 is an example of the notification email you will receive. **Note:** You will not be able to log in to Harris CareTracker until you have received the notification email. It may take up to 24 hours for your Harris CareTracker training company to be created and to receive the notification.

Hello cengage238032,

Your training company has been successfully created. Log in and begin using CareTracker's training environment at training.CareTracker.com

Harris CareTracker has worked with tens of thousands of physicians to create healthier practices and healthier patients. The training environment is a lite version of the complete practice management and EMR solutions we offer to our customers. We look forward to working with you in the future.

Sincerely,
The Harris CareTracker Practice Management and EMR Team

Courtesy of Harris Care Tracker PM and EMR

FIGURE 1-9 Welcome Login Email

Note: On subsequent logins, you will receive a *Message from webpage* that says "There is no Operator Batch Control for this Group". Click "OK" and a dialog box called *Operator Encounter Batch Control* will display when you first sign in. Close out of this box by clicking the *Save* button and then clicking the "X" at the top right of the box (Figure 1-10).

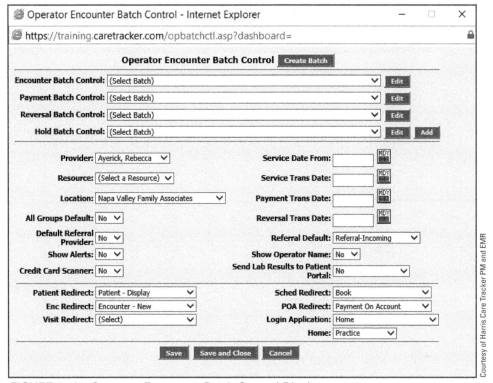

FIGURE 1-10   *Operator Encounter Batch Control Display*

 CRITICAL THINKING   Now that you have completed your Chapter 1 activities, how did the challenge put forth in the Real-World Connection apply? Did you carefully read and implement all of the directions when setting up your computer for the first time? Were you able to successfully create your Harris CareTracker training company? Elaborate on your successes and any challenges you encountered.

Introduction to Harris CareTracker PM and EMR

2

Learning Objectives

1. Log in to Harris CareTracker to complete activities.
2. Use the *Help* system to become familiar with key features of Harris CareTracker PM and EMR and to access step-by-step instructions on using each aspect of the system to quickly and successfully complete required tasks.
3. Explain the purpose and location of the *Main Menu*, *Navigation*, *Home*, and *Dashboard*.
4. Identify *Administration* features and functions for *Practice Management* and Electronic Medical Records.
5. Use the *Message Center* components for appropriate EHR tasks.

Real-World Connection

Prior to using the EHR software in our practice, medical assistants are required to become certified as "Super Users" of Harris CareTracker PM and EMR. The training that employees receive to obtain this status is similar to the training you will receive throughout this workbook. This chapter introduces you to the *Help* system, which features a variety of video links and written training materials that elaborate on the training outlined in each chapter. Employees who utilize these materials typically perform at a higher level than those who do not. Your challenge is to utilize the *Help* materials to enhance the training process and expand your knowledge.

ALERT! Due to the evolving nature and continuous upgrades of real-world EMRs such as this one, as you log in and work in your student version of Harris CareTracker there may be a slightly different look to your live screen from the screenshots provided in this workbook.

When prompted, follow the instructions given in the text to complete the activities.

Before you begin the activities in this chapter, review the Best Practices list on page xiv of this workbook. These Best Practices are provided to help you complete work quickly and accurately in Harris CareTracker PM and EMR. Review these Best Practices periodically so that they become second nature.

LOG IN TO HARRIS CARETRACKER

Learning Objective 1: Log in to Harris CareTracker to complete activities.

Activity 2-1

Log in to Harris CareTracker PM and EMR

There are system readiness requirements that must be met before logging in to Harris CareTracker. These instructions are found in Chapter 1, Activities 1-1 through 1-8 and must be completed prior to working in Harris CareTracker. You must "clear your cache" (Activity 1-6) before logging in for each session.

In Chapter 1, Activity 1-9, you registered your credentials and created your Harris CareTracker PM and EMR training company using your preassigned user name located on the inside front cover of your book and the password you created when setting up your training company. Before beginning the activities, clear your cache. If you are using a personal computer (PC), only work in Internet Explorer 11®. Use Safari® for iPad®. Once the cache has been cleared, you may continue by logging in to your student version of Harris CareTracker.

1. Go to *http://www.cengage.com/CareTracker*.

2. The domain is set to "Current" by default (**Figure 2-1**). Leave as is.

3. The product list is set to "Cengage Learning Harris CareTracker Simulation 1.0" by default. Leave as is.

4. In the *Username* box, enter the username preassigned to you. **Note:** Both the username and password are case sensitive.

5. In the *Password* box, enter your password you created in Chapter 1, Activity 1-9. **Note:** As noted in Chapter 1, on each subsequent login, a dialog box called *Operator Encounter Batch Control* will display when you first sign in. Close out of this box by clicking the *Save* button and then clicking the "X" at the top right of the box (refer to Figure 1-11).

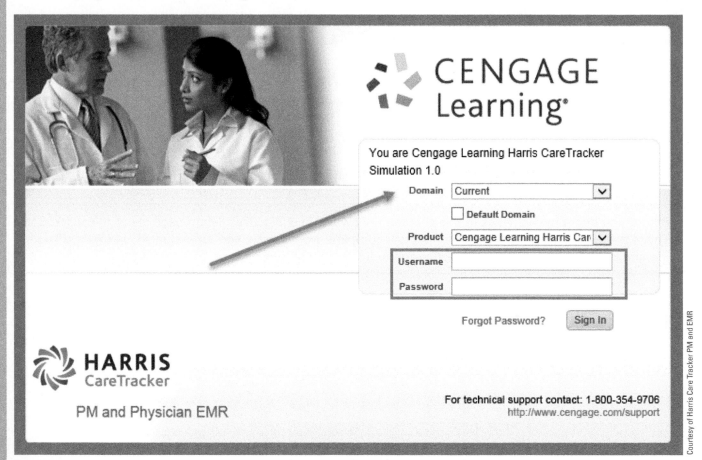

Figure 2-1   Login Screen

HELP SYSTEM

Learning Objective 2: Use the Help system to become familiar with key features of Harris CareTracker PM and EMR and to access step-by-step instructions on using each aspect of the system to quickly and successfully complete required tasks.

Activity 2-2

Recorded Training—General Navigation and Help

Harris CareTracker PM and EMR online *Help* integrates product help, recorded training sessions, live webinars, support documentation, and quick reference tools to help you learn about and use Harris CareTracker PM and EMR. The Harris CareTracker PM and EMR *Help* system offers an invaluable one-stop resource for both novice and advanced users. It is designed to familiarize the user with key features of Harris CareTracker PM and EMR, and it provides step-by-step instructions on using each aspect of the system to quickly and successfully complete required tasks.

As with all live programs, there are continual updates. The same is true for Harris CareTracker. While Harris CareTracker strives to have the most current information available in *Help*, there are instances where you may notice an update in the program that has not been updated in *Help*. This may include a reference to "Optum" PM & Physician EMR and "Ingenix." The content is the same, regardless of the title reference.

To learn more about Harris CareTracker and the *Help* features provided, click on the *General Navigation and Help System* training under the *Practice Management Recorded Training* header and view the video. The most current version of documents is always available in *Help* for easy reference. Refer back to the recorded trainings throughout your studies as needed.

1. Click on *Help.*
2. At the top of the screen, click on the *Training* button. (**Note:** The *Training* button is to the left of the *Support* button.)
3. Click on "Learn More" under *Recorded Training.*
4. Scroll down to *Practice Management.*
5. Click on the *General Navigation and Help System* topic (**Figure 2-2**).

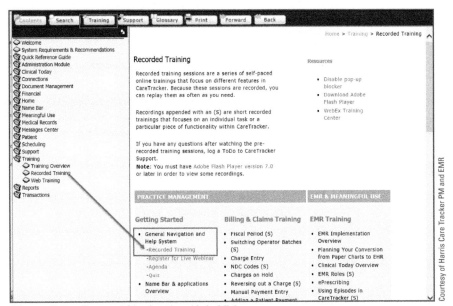

Figure 2-2   General Navigation Help Video

6. Click on the *Recorded Training* link to watch the video.

Print a screenshot taken during your viewing of the Recorded Training, label it "Activity 2-2," and place it in your assignment folder.

7. After you finish viewing the Recorded Training, click on the "X" in the upper-right corner of the *Recorded Training* box. Do <u>not</u> close out of Harris CareTracker.

Activity 2-3
Snipit (S) Fiscal Period

A "Snipit" is a short recorded training that focuses on an individual task or a particular piece of functionality within Harris CareTracker PM and EMR. Snipits are identified with an (S) following the topic header. If you have any questions after watching a Snipit (S) video, you can watch one of the longer recorded training sessions that include the topic. You will view a Snipit (S) in this activity by clicking on *Learn More* under *Recorded Training* (**Figure 2-3**).

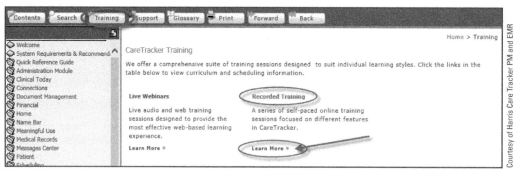

Figure 2-3   Help Snipit Learn More

1. Click on *Help* ⭕.

2. Click on the *Training* button on the toolbar.

3. Click on "Learn More" under *Recorded Training.*

4. Scroll down to the *Practice Management* section. The recorded trainings are grouped by topic area. Any training with an "(S)" at the end of the title is a Snipit training.

5. Click on the *Fiscal Period (S)* topic under "Billing & Claims Training" (**Figure 2-4**).

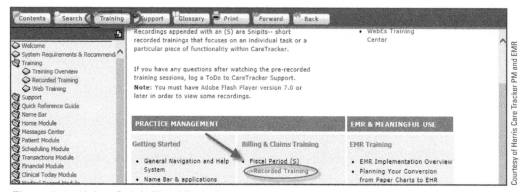

Figure 2-4   Help—Snipit Fiscal Period

6. Click on the *Recorded Training* link to watch the video.

    *   You must have Adobe Flash Player version 7.0 or later to view a *Snipit (S)* recording. The first time you view a recorded training you may be prompted to download and install the Adobe Flash Player if you do not already have it installed.

    *   If you find that the *Recording Training* or *Snipits (S)* are running slow or freezing, you may need to log out, clear your cache, and log back in to begin your activities.

Print the Snipit Fiscal Period screen, label it "Activity 2-3," and place it in your assignment folder.

MAIN MENU AND NAVIGATION

Learning Objective 3: Explain the purpose and location of the Main Menu, Navigation, Home, and Dashboard.

There are three applications contained in the *Home* module; *Dashboard*, *Messages*, and *News*. (**Figure 2-5**). There are also three tabs: *Practice*, *Management*, and *Meaningful Use.* Your Harris CareTracker PM and EMR role determines which applications you can access. Your *Home* screen is set to default to the *Home > Dashboard > Practice* screen.

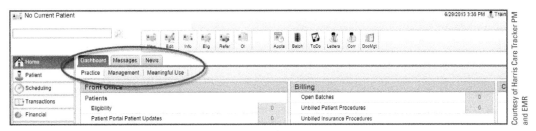

Figure 2-5   Home Application Tabs

Home Overview

In Harris CareTracker PM and EMR, the *Dashboard* is where you find your quick links to front office, billing, and clinical functions and features. The *Messages* application is a communication tool used to manage *ToDos*, mail messages, and faxes. The *News* application provides the ability to post messages to patients and employees, ensuring that important information is made available in a timely manner. In your student version of Harris CareTracker, you can visit the *News* application for important messages from Cengage and Harris CareTracker, but you will not be able to post messages yourself (**Figure 2-6**).

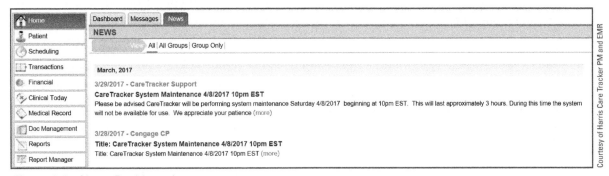

Figure 2-6   News Dashboard

Dashboard Overview

In Harris CareTracker PM and EMR, the *Dashboard* is considered "information central." At a quick glance, you can see a summary of what activity has taken place in your practice, and you can also see what key indicators need to be addressed, such as inactive claims. The *Dashboard* is divided into three tabs: *Practice*, *Management*, and *Meaningful Use* (**Figure 2-7**).

- *Practice.* The *Practice* tab contains *Front Office*, *Billing*, and *Clinical* application summaries.
- *Management.* The *Management* tab includes the practice's financial and management functions.
- *Meaningful Use.* The *Meaningful Use* tab measures and tracks a provider's progress toward meeting each of the Meaningful Use requirements and to qualify for the Medicaid and Medicare EHR incentive programs.

Courtesy of Harris Care Tracker PM and EMR

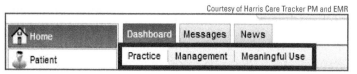

Figure 2-7   Dashboard Tabs

ADMINISTRATION FEATURES AND FUNCTIONS

Learning Objective 4: Identify Administration features and functions for Practice Management and Electronic Medical Records.

The *Administration* module contains the *Administration* application, which is divided into three tabs: *Practice*, *Clinical*, and *Setup*. Each tab is organized into sections containing links to other applications in Harris CareTracker PM.

Practice—Daily Administration

Although there are numerous features in the *Administration* module, we will focus on the applications you will use during the course of your training relative to practice management.

Activity 2-4
Open a New Fiscal Year

Working in the correct fiscal period is crucial in the electronic health record. Transactions and entries are permanently linked to a fiscal period and must be accurate. You must define the fiscal periods for your practice before any charges or payments are entered into Harris CareTracker PM and EMR. You can manage the practice's financials by opening and closing each fiscal period. You can post financials to multiple open periods, but you cannot post financials or create a batch for a closed period. The fiscal period and year you are working in displays in all financial transaction applications, such as *Charge*, *Bulk Charges*, and *Payments on Account*. All reports are linked to the established fiscal periods, not the periods of the calendar year.

Depending on when you begin using this workbook, you may be required to change the fiscal year in addition to opening fiscal periods. This activity instructs you how to open a new fiscal year.

1. Click the *Administration* module. Harris CareTracker PM displays the *Practice* tab.

2. Under the *System Administration* column, in the *Financial* section, click the *Open/Close Period* link (**Figure 2-8**). Harris CareTracker PM displays all of your fiscal periods for the current fiscal year.

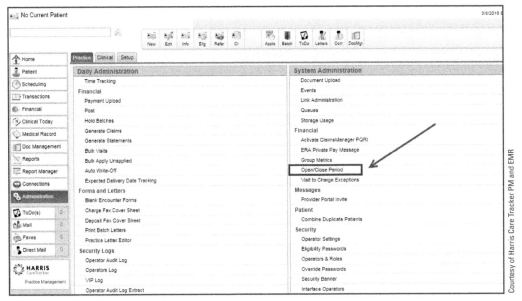

Figure 2-8   Open/Close Period

3. Enter the year in the *Fiscal Year* field. **Note:** If the *Fiscal Year* already displays for the current year you are working, move on to the next step. If you need to change the fiscal year, enter the current year and click *Go.*

4. To open a fiscal year for all groups within your company, select "Y" from the *All Groups* drop-down menu and then click *Go* (**Figure 2-9**).

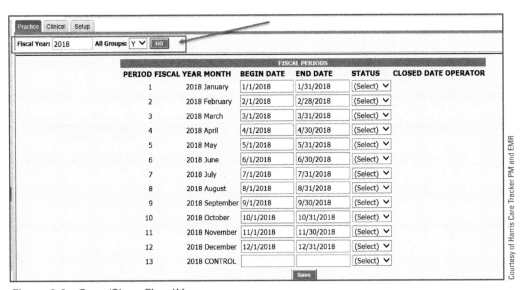

Figure 2-9   Open/Close Fiscal Year

5. By default, the beginning and end date of each period is set to the first and last days of the month. Leave as is.

6. Continue with Activity 2-5 to open a new fiscal period.

📄 **Print the Open Fiscal Year screen, label it "Activity 2-4," and place it in your assignment folder.**

Activity 2-5

Open a Fiscal Period

On the first day of a new period, the practice administrator must change the status of the period to *Open* to begin posting financials to that period. You can also open a period prior to the first day of the period. It is typical for a practice to have multiple periods open.

You will have to open periods while working throughout the text to reflect the current date(s) of the activities you are working in.

> **ALERT!** Do <u>not</u> close a fiscal period unless instructed to do so.

1. Continue from Activity 2-4. If you had already logged out:

   a. Click the *Administration* module. Harris CareTracker PM displays the *Practice* tab.

   b. Under *System Administration/Financial*, click the *Open/Close Period* link. Harris CareTracker PM displays all of your fiscal periods for the current fiscal year.

   c. For multigroup companies, select "Y" from the *All Groups* drop-down list and then click *Go* to open a fiscal period for all groups in the company.

2. From the list in the *Status* column, use the drop down and select "OPEN" for the period you want to open. Open the period (month/year) you are currently working in (for example, if the day you complete this activity is January 20, 2018, you would open fiscal period January 2018). **Note**: As you continue your work/activities in Harris CareTracker, you may need to open additional fiscal periods as well. Refer to this activity throughout the text when you need to open additional fiscal periods.

3. Click *Save*. You can now create batches and post financials for this period (**Figure 2-10**).

	PERIOD	FISCAL YEAR	MONTH	BEGIN DATE	END DATE	STATUS	CLOSED DATE	OPERATOR
	1	2017	January	1/1/2017	1/31/2017	(Select)		
	2	2017	February	2/1/2017	2/28/2017	(Select)		
	3	2017	March	3/1/2017	3/31/2017	(Select)		
EXISTS	4	2017	April	4/1/2017	4/30/2017	OPEN		Jasmine Brady
	5	2017	May	5/1/2017	5/31/2017	(Select)		
	6	2017	June	6/1/2017	6/30/2017	(Select)		
	7	2017	July	7/1/2017	7/31/2017	(Select)		
	8	2017	August	8/1/2017	8/31/2017	(Select)		
	9	2017	September	9/1/2017	9/30/2017	(Select)		
	10	2017	October	10/1/2017	10/31/2017	(Select)		
	11	2017	November	11/1/2017	11/30/2017	(Select)		
	12	2017	December	12/1/2017	12/31/2017	(Select)		
	13	2017	CONTROL			(Select)		

Fiscal Year: 2017 All Groups: Y GO

Courtesy of Harris Care Tracker PM and EMR

Figure 2-10   *Fiscal Period Open*

Print the Open Fiscal Period screen, label it "Activity 2-5," and place it in your assignment folder.

TIP You will have to open/close periods while working throughout the workbook to reflect the current date(s) and activities you are working in.

 SPOTLIGHT   Warning!! Do not close a fiscal period until instructed to do so.

Activity 2-6
Change Your Password

Every operator must have a username and a password to log in to Harris CareTracker PM and EMR. You are required to change your password every 90 days. Harris CareTracker PM and EMR reminds users seven days before their password expires and gives you the option of changing the password at that time. If your password expires, you can reset it without having to log a *ToDo* to *Support*. You can also use *Operator Settings* to change your password at any time after you begin using Harris CareTracker PM and EMR, even prior to being required to by the system.

 PROFESSIONALISM CONNECTION

The Harris CareTracker PM and EMR software allows management to track where you have been in the system. Never give anyone your password! If someone other than you uses your sign-in to view a patient's record, there is no way to prove that it was not you. If anyone asks for your password, remind him or her that it is against company policy to share passwords.

1. Click the *Administration* module. The application displays the *Practice* tab.

2. Under the *System Administration* column, in the *Security* section, click the *Operator Settings* link (**Figure 2-11**). Harris CareTracker PM and EMR launches the *Operator Settings* application.

3. In the *Old Password* box, enter your current password (the one you created in Activity 1-9).

4. In the *New Password* field, enter your new password (enter a personal password you will remember). Record your username and new password for future reference:

   a. Username: _____

   b. New Password: _____

   • The new password must meet the following criteria:

   • The new password must differ from your old password by at least one character.

   • The new password must consist of at least eight characters.

   • At least one of the eight characters must be a capital letter and at least one must be a number; for example: "Password5."

5. In the *Verify Password* box, reenter your new password.

6. From the *Question* list, select a security question.

7. In the *Answer* box, enter the answer to the security question.

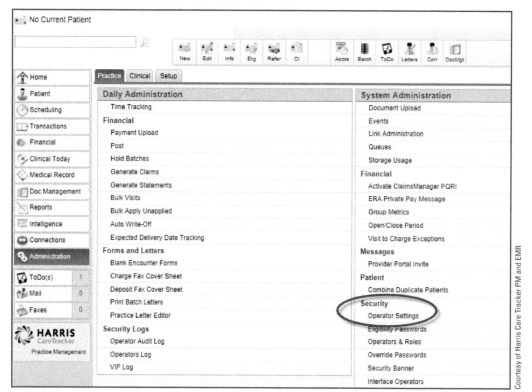

Figure 2-11   *Operator Settings*

8. In the *Phone* and *Email* fields, enter your phone number and email address. It is important to keep this contact information up to date because it is used by *Support* to follow up on support issues or *ToDos* (see **Figure 2-12**).

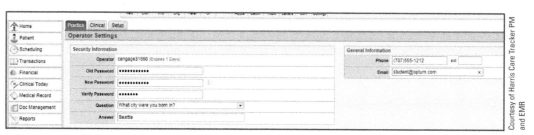

Figure 2-12   *Change Password Screen*

9. Click *Save*, and you will receive a *Success* pop-up box. Click *Close* on the pop-up box.

🖨 **Print the Change Your Password screen, label it "Activity 2-6," and place it in your assignment folder.**

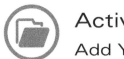

Activity 2-7
Add Your Name as Operator

All Harris CareTracker PM and EMR operators are set up with a user profile based on their responsibilities and duties in a practice. An operator's privileges in Harris CareTracker PM and EMR are determined by the *Role(s)* and *Override(s)* assigned to his or her profile. Roles determine which Harris CareTracker PM and EMR modules and applications an operator can access. Overrides are used either to restrict an operator's access to a certain application and functionality or to grant an operator additional privileges that may not be included in his or her role. For example, if an operator needs access to only one application within the *Financial* module, you could add an override to the operator's profile to allow him or her to access just a particular financial application.

In order to provide a customized user experience, you will now add your name as operator. This also helps easily identify your "training company" operator name as user.

1. Click the *Administration* module. The application displays the *Practice* tab.

2. Under the *Security* header, click the *Operators & Roles* link. The application displays the *Group Operators* list.

3. Click on your operator name. The information will display below your operator name.

4. In the *Name* section:

    a. Skip the *Title* box (not used for operators).

    b. In the *First Name* box, enter your first name.

    c. Skip the *Middle* name box (not used for operators).

    d. In the *Last Name* box, enter your last name.

5. Click *Save*. The application updates your operator name.

6. Log out of Harris CareTracker, and then log back in. Your name will now be listed as the operator (**Figure 2-13**).

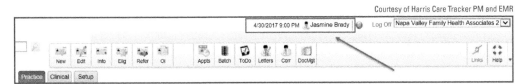

Figure 2-13   Add Your Name as Operator

Print the Updated Operator Name screen, label it "Activity 2-7," and place it in your assignment folder.

 SPOTLIGHT   The maximum idle time in Harris CareTracker PM is 180 minutes. For security reasons, it is best practice to keep the idle time short, such as 5–10 minutes. The time zone defaults to Eastern Standard Time (EST) if no time zone is set for the operator. Refer to *Help* for instructions to adjust your idle time and time zone.

Activity 2-8
Add Item(s) to a Quick Picks List

Throughout Harris CareTracker PM and EMR, drop-down lists are available from which you can select field-specific data to help create a more efficient workflow, known as *Quick Picks*. Options available in a drop-down list are built for each practice and are group specific. Your practice can build drop-down options for locations, employers, insurance companies, and financial transactions.

In order for certain data fields to be available as you work in Harris CareTracker PM and EMR, they need to be added to your "quick picks" list. You can add or remove options from a drop-down list in the *Quick Pick Setup* application.

1. Click the *Administration* module, and then click the *Setup* tab.

2. Under the *Financial* header, click the *Quick Picks* link (**Figure 2-14**). Harris CareTracker PM and EMR launches the *Quick Picks* application.

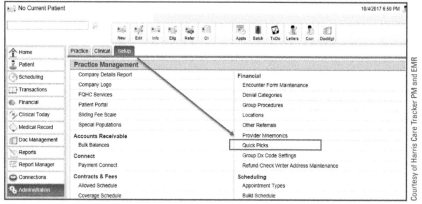

Figure 2-14   Quick Picks Link

3. From the *Screen Type* drop-down list, select the quick picks list to which you want to add an item (select "Form Letters"). The application displays the "quick picks list."

4. Verify that the item you want to add is not already included in the current "quick picks" list.

5. Enter the item you want to add in the *Search* box (enter "New") and then click the *Search* icon. The application displays a search window containing a list of possible matches (**Figure 2-15**). Click on the

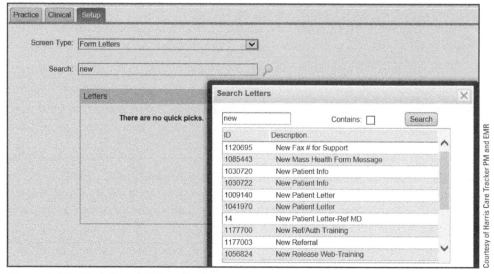

Figure 2-15   New Referral Form Letter

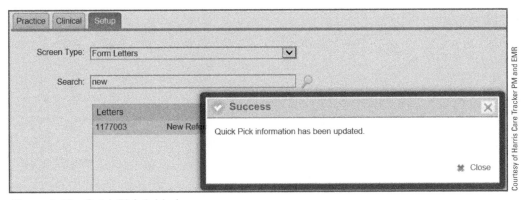

Figure 2-16   Quick Pick Added

desired result to select it (select "New Referral"). The application closes the search window and adds the data as an option in the list (**Figure 2-16**).

6. Click on "X" or "Close" to close out of the "Success" dialog box.

💾 **Print the Quick Picks screen, label it "Activity 2-8," and place it in your assignment folder.**

THE MESSAGE CENTER

Learning Objective 5: Use the Message Center components for appropriate EHR tasks.

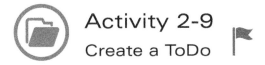

Activity 2-9
Create a ToDo

The *ToDo* application is Harris CareTracker PM and EMR's internal messaging system that allows you to assign administrative and patient-related tasks within your practice as well as communicate with the Harris CareTracker PM and EMR support team. You will know you have an open *ToDo* if a number appears next to the *ToDo* link in the left navigation pane. In the *ToDo* application, you can review each *ToDo* that has been sent to you, reply to a *ToDo*, transfer a *ToDo*, take ownership of a *ToDo*, or close a *ToDo*. The application is updated in real time.

1. Click the *Home* module, and then click the *Messages* tab. The *Messages* application displays all of your open *ToDo*(s).

2. Click on the *ToDo* 🗒 icon on the *Name Bar*. The application displays the *New ToDo* window (**Figure 2-17**).

3. Leave the *Macro Name* blank.

4. By default, the *From* list displays your operator name.

5. In the *To* list, click the required options. The *To* list includes the categories described in **Figure 2-18**. Select "Operator" in the first field and "Self" in the second field.

6. If you are sending a *ToDo* to a patient, enter his or her full or partial last name in the *Patient* box (enter "Wild") and then click the *Search* 🔍 icon. When the search window opens, click on the name of the patient in the search results (search "Wild"; select "Wild, Alison").

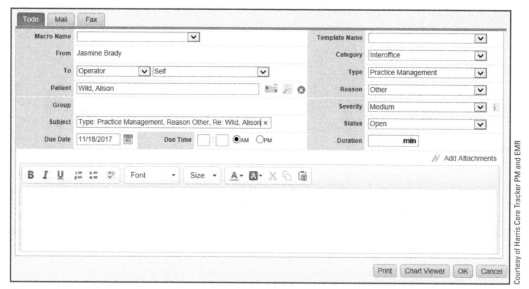

Figure 2-17   ToDo Dialog Box

TODO LIST OPTIONS

Field	Description
Operator	Enables you to select a CareTracker user from your company.
Queue	Enables you to select a work queue set up for the practice. This will redirect the ToDo to the queue. For example, you can send a ToDo to the Support queue and an operator in the queue will respond to the ToDo.
Participant	Enables you to select a participant in the ToDo. This can be a person or a queue that participated in the ToDo.

Figure 2-18   List Options for ToDo

 TIP If the *ToDo* is not patient related, you would click the *Delete* icon ✖ to remove the name from the *Patient* field. You can click the *Info* 🔳 icon to view the patient's contact information in the "At a Glance" patient information window.

7. By default, the *Subject* box displays information based on the selection in the *Type* and *Reason* lists in the right-hand column. However, you can change the subject if necessary. Leave as "Practice Management, Reason Other, Re: Wild, Alison."

8. In the *Due Date* and *Due Time* boxes, enter the date and time by which the *ToDo* should be completed. This is important to track overdue items. Leave the *Due Date* as is and in the *Due Time* enter 05:00 and then select PM.

9. Leave the *Template Name* field blank.

10. From the C*ategory* list, select the *ToDo* category (leave as "Interoffice").

11. In the *Type* list, click/confirm the type of the *ToDo* (leave as "Practice Management").

12. In the *Reason* list, click/confirm the reason for the *ToDo* (leave as "Other").

13. In the *Severity* list, select the priority level of the *ToDo* (leave as "Medium").

14. The *Status* list is set to "Open" by default. Leave as is.

15. In the *Duration* box, enter the total time spent working on the *ToDo* (enter "5").

16. In the text box, type in "Test ToDo."

17. Click *OK*. The *ToDo* will disappear and show in your *Messages Dashboard* (**Figure 2-19**).

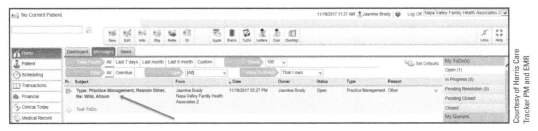

Figure 2-19   Student-Created ToDo

 Print the *Messages* dashboard with the completed *ToDo*, label it "Activity 2-9," and place it in your assignment folder.

Activity 2-10
Create a New Mail Message

The *Mail* application allows you to communicate electronically with staff members, providers in your *Provider Portal*, and patients activated in the *Patient Portal*. The mail feature works the same as other email applications, enabling you to open, view, create, send and receive, and delete messages. In addition, you can link attachments such as patient encounter notes, documents, results, referrals and authorization forms, set priorities, and more.

1. Click the *Home* module, and then click the *Messages* tab. The *Messages Center* opens and displays all of your open *ToDo*s.

2. Click *Send Mail*, located on the lower-right-side *ToDo* pane (**Figure 2-20**). The application displays the *New Mail* dialog box.

3. Leave the *Macro Name* as is: (-Select-).

4. The *From* list defaults to the operator creating the mail message and cannot be edited.

5. In the *To* field, click the *Search* icon. Harris CareTracker PM and EMR opens the *Select Operators* dialog box.

6. Place a check mark in the box by *your* login name (see example in **Figure 2-21**). **Note:** The last name field will either include your last name or your CareTracker username.

7. Click *Select*. The application closes the *Select Operators* dialog box.

8. If a patient is in context, the patient name displays in the *Patient* box. However, you can also send a mail message about a different patient by clicking the *Search* icon. For this activity, you will leave the patient field blank. If a patient is in context, click the red "x" at the end of the patient name field to remove the patient from context.

9. In the *Subject* box, enter the subject of the mail message (enter "Test Mail Message").

10. Leave the *Template Name* field blank.

11. By default, the *Severity* list displays "Medium." However, you can change the severity of the mail message if necessary. Leave as is.

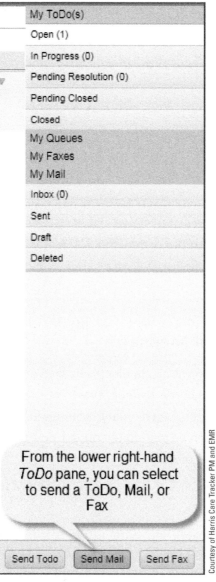

Figure 2-20   Send Mail

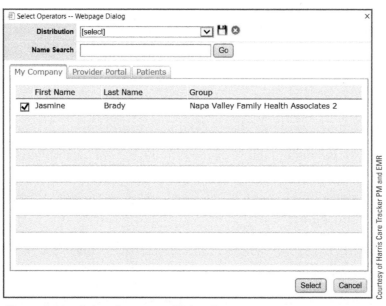

Figure 2-21   Select Operators Dialog Box

12. (FYI) To link a clinical document or chart summary, refer to the instructions in *Help*. Do not link or add any data.

13. In the message dialog box, enter the message and format the information if necessary. Enter "Test Mail Message" (**Figure 2-22**).

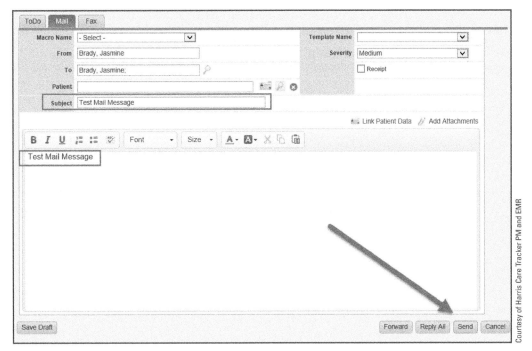

Figure 2-22   Send Test Mail Message

14. Click *Send*. If you did not want to send the message immediately you would click *Save Draft* to save the message and send later. For this activity, click *Send*.

15. To view your sent message, click the *Sent* link on the *My ToDo(s)* pane on the right side of the screen (**Figure 2-23**) or the Mail link on the left-hand side of your screen.

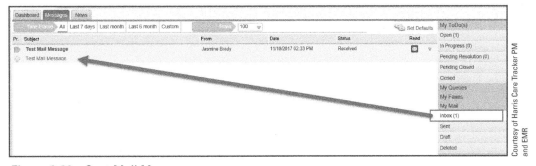

Figure 2-23   Sent Mail Message

 Print the Sent Message screen, label it "Activity 2-10," and place it in your assignment folder.

CRITICAL THINKING In the beginning of this chapter, your challenge was to utilize the *Help* materials to enhance the training process and expand your knowledge. Which features in *Help* did you access? What topics did you find most helpful? If you experienced any challenges completing the activities, did you log in to *Help* to look for support? If not, why not?

CASE STUDIES

Case Study 2-1

Create a *ToDo* for patient Harriet Oshea. (Refer to Activity 2-9 for guidance.) For this case study, enter the following text for the *ToDo*:

"Test ToDo (CS 2-1): Dr. Brockton, patient Harriet Oshea called to follow up on her joint pain. Your schedule is full the next three weeks. Would you like me to double book her this week?"

Print a copy of the screen that illustrate you created a ToDo for Harriet Oshea, label it "Case Study 2-1," and place it in your assignment folder.

Patient Demographics and Registration

Learning Objectives

1. Identify components of the Name Bar.
2. Describe the Patient Module and Demographics features in Harris CareTracker.
3. Search for a patient within Harris CareTracker PM.
4. Edit patient information in Harris CareTracker.
5. View and perform eligibility checks.

Real-World Connection

Here at NVFHA, we conduct reference checks on all job applicants who make it to a second interview. Our goal is to hire applicants who have a high capacity for "attention to detail." When entering patient demographic information in the computer, it is critical to pay attention to detail because this information impacts so many departments within our practice. If you misspell a patient's name, put in incorrect address information, or omit insurance information, it creates havoc for the clinical team searching for the patient's chart, the billing team that has to send out a second billing statement, and even the insurance company that reviews a claim for the second time. Patients are often impacted as well by these types of errors and lose confidence in the overall practice. These types of errors are costly to the practice because they increase employee hours needed to make corrections and delay reimbursement for services that affect the revenue cycle.

As you go through the activities in this chapter, pay particular attention to your ability to enter information correctly. If you struggle in this area, you may want to slow down a bit and make certain that you are entering the correct information the first time around.

Keep this information in mind as you begin your activities. At the end of the chapter, you will be asked to summarize your experience. Are you up for the challenge? Let's get started!

Before you begin the activities in this chapter, refresh your memory on working with Harris CareTracker by referring back to the Best Practices list on page xiv of this workbook. Following best practices will help you complete work quickly and accurately.

NAME BAR

Learning Objective 1: Identify components of the Name Bar.

The *Name Bar*, located across the top of the Harris CareTracker window, provides quick access to the most frequently used Harris CareTracker applications (**Figure 3-1**). A quick reference guide to the various applications launched from the *Name Bar* illustrates each button and a description of the function (**Figure 3-2**). The *Name Bar* allows you to pull a patient into context to perform specific tasks. A patient is "in context" when his or her information appears in the *Name* list and *ID* box, as illustrated on the *Name Bar* picture.

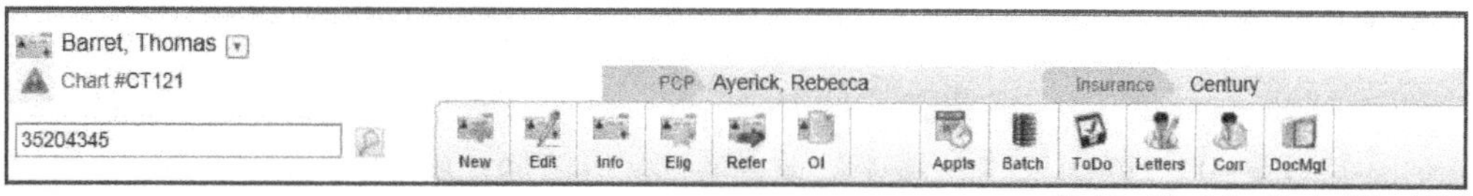

Figure 3-1   Name Bar

Courtesy of Harris Care Tracker PM and EMR

NAME BAR	
Button	**Description**
Search	Pulls patients into context by Harris CareTracker PM and EMR ID number, chart number, claim ID, or last name. Enter the patient's first name, last name, or at least three letters of each name to display the Advanced Search dialog box that enables you to select a patient.
Alert	Displays the Patient Alerts window. The Patient Alerts window notifies the operator when key information is missing from a patient's demographics or if any problems exist with the patient's account.
Edit	Launches the Demographics application in edit mode for the patient in context.
New	Launches the Demographics application, enabling you to register a new patient in Harris CareTracker PM and EMR.
Info	Displays a read only summary of the patient's information, including address, contact information, family members, balance information, insurance, etc.
Elig	Displays a history of eligibility checks and enables you to perform an individual electronic eligibility check to ensure that the patient is covered by the insurance company listed as the primary insurance.
Refer	Launches the Referral/Authorization application.
Appts	Displays a list of upcoming patient appointments. In addition, you can view and confirm an appointment, check in/check out a patient, print the encounter form, and perform various other tasks pertaining to the appointment.
OI	Displays information pertaining to dates of service. For example, you can obtain information such as associated procedures, financial transactions and claim activity, and make financial transactions such as payments, adjustments, refunds, and more.
Batch	Launches the Batch application, allowing you to create a new batch to enter charges and post payments and adjustments. In addition, you can also set up personal settings when using Harris CareTracker PM and EMR. For example, the main application to launch when logged on to Harris CareTracker PM and EMR.
ToDo	Launches the Harris CareTracker PM and EMR messaging tool, allowing you to communicate with other staff and the Harris CareTracker PM and EMR Support Department.
Letters	Generates and prints letters to send to a patient.
Corr	Displays a queue of letters generated and enables you to print the letters to send to patients.

Figure 3-2   Description of Name Bar Applications

Courtesy of Harris Care Tracker PM and EMR

DEMOGRAPHICS

Learning Objective 2: Describe the Patient Module and Demographics features in Harris CareTracker.

The *Demographics* application in the *Patient* module is where new patients are registered and added into the Harris CareTracker PM and EMR system. A patient's record will contain basic identifying information and is where pertinent health insurance information is captured. Demographics in the medical field can be described as defining or descriptive information on the patient (e.g., name, address, phone number[s], sex, insurance information, DOB [age], ethnicity).

SEARCH FOR A PATIENT

Learning Objective 3: Search for a patient within Harris CareTracker PM.

Activity 3-1

Search for a Patient by Name (currently in the database)

To search for patient Alison Wild by name:

1. In the *ID* search box on the *Name Bar*, enter the first three letters of the patient's last name ["Wil"], and hit [Enter] (**Figure 3-3**). The pop-up will list any patient matching your search criteria. Click on patient "Alison Wild." If you receive a pop-up asking if you want to navigate away from this page (**Figure 3-4**), select *OK* and Harris CareTracker PM will launch the *Patient Demographics* page, displaying the patient's demographics screen.

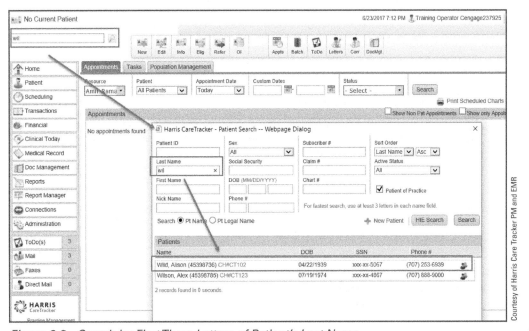

Figure 3-3   Search by First Three Letters of Patient's Last Name

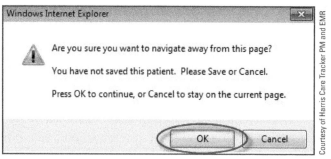

Figure 3-4   Leave This Page Pop-Up Message

TIP An alternate method to search for existing patients is:

1. Remove a patient in context by clicking on the drop-down list at the end of the patient's name (**Figure 3-5**) and select "None." The name in the patient field will be removed and "No Current Patient" will display.

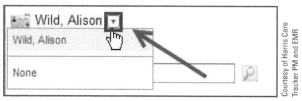

Figure 3-5   Remove Patient from Context Drop-Down

2. With "No Current Patient" in the *ID* search box, click on the *Search* 🔍 icon, which will bring up the *Patient Search* box.

3. In the *Patient Search* box, enter at least three letters of the patient's last ("Wil") and first name ("Ali"). A previous name such as a maiden name or an alias cannot be used to search for a patient.

4. Click the *Search* button. The *Patient Search* box displays a list of patients that match the information entered (see Figure 3-3), along with the patient ID and chart number.

5. Click the *Family* icon 👥 to view the patient's family members registered in Harris CareTracker PM and EMR (if applicable).

6. Verify the "second identifier" such as DOB or last four numbers of the Social Security number, and then click the specific name to launch the patient into context (see Figure 3-3).

2. Record the patient's ID number, chart number, and Social Security number for additional activities related to searching for a patient. _____

3. Click the specific name to launch the patient into context.

🖥 **Print the Patient Demographics screen, label it "Activity 3-1," and place it in your assignment folder.**

PROFESSIONALISM CONNECTION

Start every conversation with a patient either over the phone or in person by asking for a minimum of two identifiers. Most offices have patients state their first and last names followed by their birth date. This helps to confirm that you are in the correct chart and reduces the risk of documenting in the wrong chart.

Activity 3-2
Searching for a Patient by ID Number

You now have successfully searched for a patient and know the patient's ID number, chart number, Social Security number, and claim number (if applicable) from the record provided. Using that information, practice searching for the same patient using alternative methods.

1. With no patient in context, in the *ID* search box (see Figure 3-3), enter patient Alison Wild's *ID number* (using the *ID number* obtained from the patient search in Activity 3-1). (**Note:** New ID numbers are assigned to patients for each student version of Harris CareTracker; therefore, patient ID numbers will vary by student.)

2. Hit [Enter]. The patient with the corresponding *ID number* launches into context.

3. You can also perform a search by patient *ID number* by clicking the *Search* icon. In the *Patient Search* box, enter the *Patient ID* number. A list of patients that match the information entered will pop up.

🖫 **Print a screenshot of the Search Results screen for Alison Wild, label it "Activity 3-2," and place it in your assignment folder.**

Activity 3-3
Searching for a Patient by Chart Number

You may also search for a patient by chart number. Typically, the chart number and the Harris CareTracker PM and EMR ID are the same. However, if the practice files paper charts by chart number, Harris CareTracker PM and EMR can assign chart numbers based on your medical record number. In your student version, the chart number and ID number are different for existing patients. New patients will have the same chart number and ID number. (**Note:** If your practice has electronically converted patient demographics to Harris CareTracker PM and EMR from another practice management system, the chart number will be the patient's ID number from your legacy practice management system.)

1. With no patient in context, click the *Search* 🔍 icon; it will take you to the *Patient Search* pop-up box where you will need to enter the patient's *Chart Number*.

2. Enter the chart number of patient Alison Wild (CT102) and click *Search* (**Figure 3-6**).

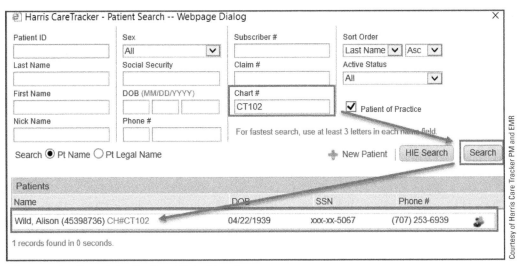

Figure 3-6   Search by Patient Chart Number

Print a screenshot of the Search Results screen, label it "Activity 3-3," and place it in your assignment folder.

3. Click directly on the patient's name with the corresponding *Chart Number* to launch him or her into context. (**Note:** It may take a few moments for Harris CareTracker to "search" and populate the patient demographics.)

Activity 3-4
Searching for a Patient by Social Security Number (SSN)

1. With no patient in context, click the *Search* 🔍 icon.

2. In the *Patient Search* pop-up box, enter the last four digits of patient Alison Wild's *Social Security* number (5067) obtained in Activity 3-1 (**Figure 3-7**), and hit [Enter] (or click on the *Search* button).

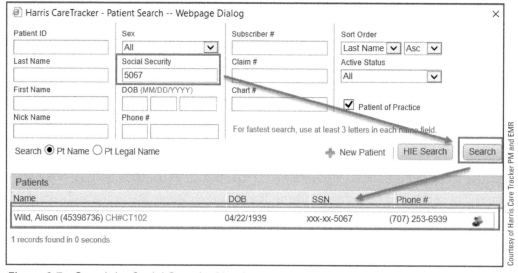

Figure 3-7 Search by Social Security Number

 Print a screenshot of the Patient Search pop-up screen, label it "Activity 3-4," and place it in your assignment folder.

3. Click on the corresponding patient (see Figure 3-7).

4. The application pulls the patient into context.

 PROFESSIONALISM CONNECTION

Registration is often the first encounter patients experience during the initial office visit. The medical assistant responsible for this task sets the tone for the remainder of the visit. If the medical assistant is curt and unfriendly, the patient may feel uneasy and may be tempted to leave; however, if the medical assistant is friendly and courteous, the patient will likely feel more at ease and comfortable proceeding with the remainder of the visit. Consider how your role as biller and coder can make a positive impact on patient relations.

EDIT PATIENT INFORMATION

Learning Objective 4: Edit patient information in Harris CareTracker.

Activity 3-5
Edit Patient Information

It is important that all patients in the Harris CareTracker PM and EMR have complete and correct demographic information such as name, contact information, date of birth, insurance and employer information, primary (PCP) and referring provider, and more. This information is required to ensure proper treatment as well as to facilitate billing. If you are registering a new patient, always search the database to be certain that the patient has never been registered. Use two patient identifiers when searching to avoid creating a duplicate account.

It is important to verify accuracy and update information when a patient schedules an appointment or checks in for an appointment. This makes the treatment process faster and avoids unnecessary complications in billing due to outdated information (**Figure 3-8**).

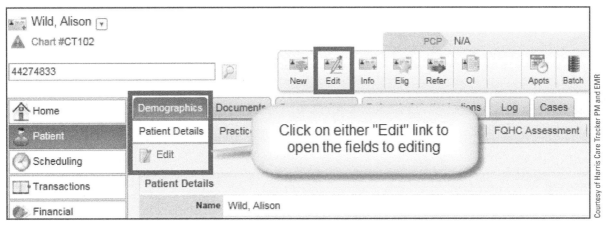

Figure 3-8   Edit Patient Information Tab

 TIP Navigate through each field by pressing the [Tab] key and Harris CareTracker PM and EMR will automatically format the entry, regardless of the way it is entered. For example, by tabbing through the *First Name* and *Last Name* boxes, Harris CareTracker PM and EMR automatically applies title case to the name, meaning the first letter of each name is capitalized. To navigate back to a field, press [SHIFT+TAB].

Search the existing database to confirm that the patient (Alison Wild) has previously been registered. After confirming she is in the system, review the demographics screen to see if all information is correct and complete. You will notice that the PCP has not yet been entered for Alison. You will edit her demographics to add Dr. Raman as her PCP.

To edit patient demographics:

1. With patient Alison Wild in context, click on the *Patient* module > *Demographics* tab (**Figure 3-9**).

2. Click on the *Edit* icon in the *Name Bar*.

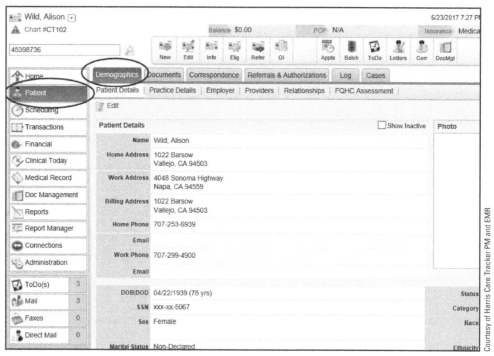

Figure 3-9 Demographics Tab

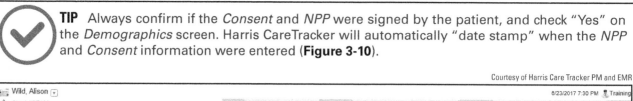

TIP Always confirm if the *Consent* and *NPP* were signed by the patient, and check "Yes" on the *Demographics* screen. Harris CareTracker will automatically "date stamp" when the *NPP* and *Consent* information were entered (**Figure 3-10**).

Courtesy of Harris Care Tracker PM and EMR

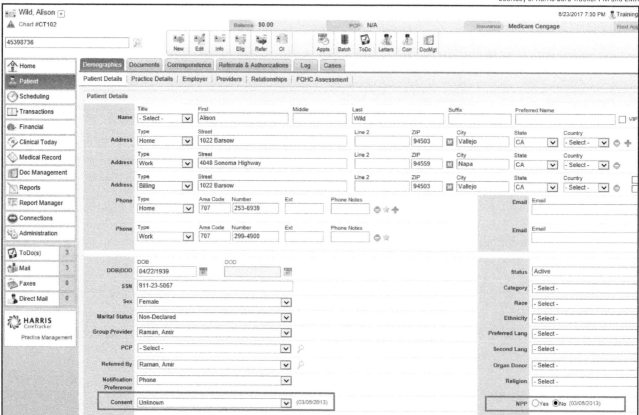

Figure 3-10 New Patient Demographic Screen with Consent and NPP Fields Highlighted

3. Scroll down the demographics page and you will note that the *PCP* (primary care provider) has not been selected. It is best practice to update any missing information when you access a patient's chart. Select the *PCP* for the patient noted on the registration form from the drop-down list. Select "Dr. Amir Raman." (**Note:** If you were searching for a provider who is not on the list, you would click the *Search* icon to the right of the field (**Figure 3-11**), type in as much information as you have (minimally last name and state), and search for the provider. You would normally select the provider listed on the patient registration form.

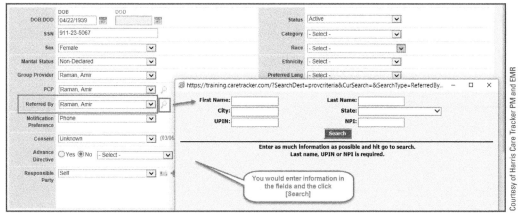

Figure 3-11   PCP Search Icon

4. *Group Provider.* Confirm from the demographics screen that Dr. Raman has been selected as the *Group Provider.*

5. Scroll down the screen and click *Save.*

6. (Informational) The *Insurance Plan*(s) section is where you update patient insurance information (**Figures 3-12** and **3-13**). (**Note:** You will refer back to this later in the workbook.)

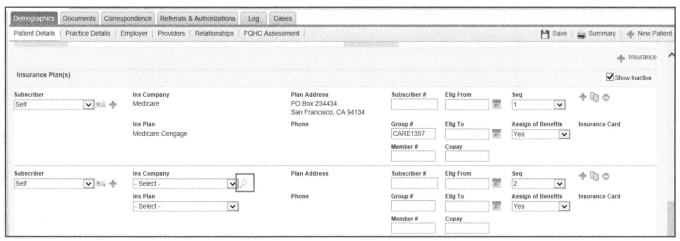

Figure 3-12   Subscriber Field Options

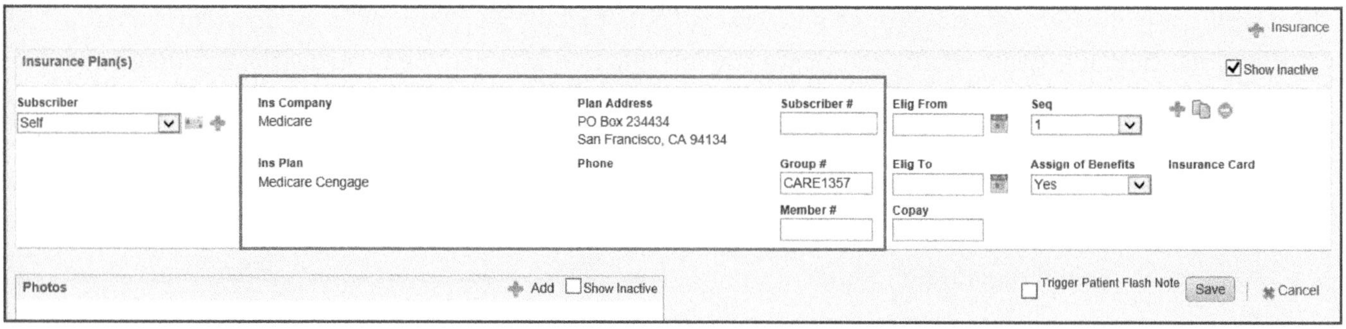

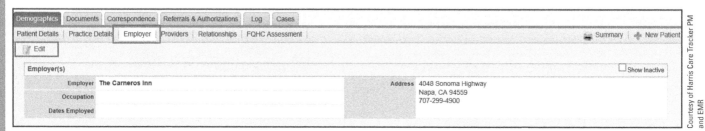

Figure 3-13 Select Subscriber's Insurance Plan

7. (Informational) The *Employer* tab under *Demographics* is where you update patient employer information (**Figure 3-14**).

Figure 3-14 Employer Field in Patient Demographics Screen

8. After updating patient registration, you may receive a pop-up alert advising you of missing information (**Figure 3-15**).

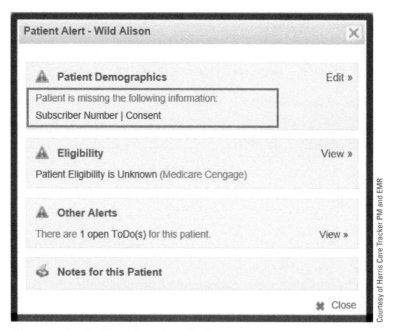

Figure 3-15 Patient Alerts Pop-Up Box

🖴 **Print the completed Demographics Summary (or take a screenshot), label it "Activity 3-5," and place it in your assignment folder.**

TIP In order to complete the remainder of the demographics information, you would click *Edit* and continue the full registration process for any missing information. It is important to know that all fields should be completed, although they are not required. The pop-up will also alert you to missing information such as primary location (should be "Napa Valley Family Associates [NVFA]"), primary language, secondary language, ethnicity, race, organ donor status, and religion. To complete these fields, with the patient in context, you would click on the *Patient* module. Select the *Patient Details* tab under the *Demographics* tab. Click on *Edit* above the *Patient Details* screen, complete the information, then hit *Save*. There are additional fields in the *Patient Details* box, which may or may not be used by the practice.

Activity 3-6
Print the Patient Demographics Report

Medical practices may find it useful to print a patient's demographic report for a variety of reasons. Some practices will give a copy of the printed report to a patient at check-in to verify information and to make any necessary corrections/updates. Following this workflow will help identify inconsistencies between the patient information and information stored in your practice management software.

1. Pull a patient into context (Alison Wild).

2. Click the *Patient* module. Harris CareTracker PM and EMR displays the *Demographics* tab.

3. Click the *Print* icon in the upper-right corner of the *Demographics* page (next to the *Summary* link). Harris CareTracker PM displays the *Print* dialog box (**Figure 3-16**). (**Note:** It may take a little time to generate the report.)

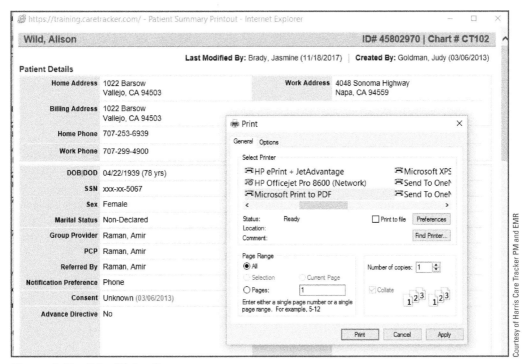

Figure 3-16   Print Dialog Box

4. Select your preferences and then click *Print* (Figure 3-17).

Wild, Alison   ID# 45802970 | Chart # CT102

Last Modified By: Brady, Jasmine (11/18/2017)   **Created By:** Goldman, Judy (03/06/2013)

Patient Details

Home Address	1022 Barsow Vallejo, CA 94503	**Work Address**	4048 Sonoma Highway Napa, CA 94559
Billing Address	1022 Barsow Vallejo, CA 94503		
Home Phone	707-253-6939	**Email**	
Work Phone	707-299-4900	**Email**	
DOB|DOD	04/22/1939 (78 yrs)	**Status**	Active
SSN	xxx-xx-5067	**Category**	
Sex	Female	**Race**	
Marital Status	Non-Declared	**Ethnicity**	
Group Provider	Raman, Amir	**Preferred Lang**	
PCP	Raman, Amir	**Second Lang**	
Referred By	Raman, Amir	**Organ Donor**	
Notification Preference	Phone	**Religion**	
Consent	Unknown (03/06/2013)	**NPP**	No (03/06/2013)
Advance Directive	No	**Notes**	

Practice   Clinical

Responsible Party   Wild, Alison (Self)

Insurance Plan(s)

Subscriber	Company Plan	Plan Address Phone	Subscriber # Group # Member #	Elig From Elig To Copay	Seq Assign Of Benefits Insurance Card
Self (Entity)	Medicare Medicare Cengage	PO Box 234434 San Francisco, CA 94134 CARE1357			1 Yes

Practice Details

Chart #	CT102	**Patient of Practice**	Yes
HIE Consent	Unknown (03/06/2013)	**Hold Statements**	No
Primary Location		**Exempt from EMR Reports**	No

Patient Portal

Status	The Patient Portal is not available for this group.

Practice Defined Patient Details

FQHC Population		**IIS Reminder Consent**
IIS Protection Indicator		**IIS Registry Status**
IIS Mothers Maiden Name		

Employer(s)

Employer	**The Carneros Inn**	**Address**

Figure 3-17   *Patient Summary Printout for Alison Wild (continues)*

4048 Sonoma Highway
Napa, CA 94559
707-299-4900

Occupation	Dates Employed

Providers

Raman, Amir PCP
Internal Medicine
101 Vine Street
Napa,CA -94558
707-555-1212 | 707-555-1214 (Fax)

Relationships

There are currently no relationships for this patient.

Emergency Contacts

There are currently no emergency contacts for this patient.

Pharmacies

There are currently no pharmacies for this patient.

Attorneys

There are currently no attorneys for this patient.

Schools

There are currently no schools for this patient.

FQHC Assessment

No Assessment information for this patient.

Figure 3-17   Patient Summary Printout for Alison Wild (continued)

Print the Patient Summary Printout, label it "Activity 3-6," and place it in your assignment folder.

PROFESSIONALISM CONNECTION

Patients may become frustrated when they are asked if there have been any changes since the last office visit. Some individuals may even become aggravated when you ask to see their insurance card. This is particularly true when the patient just had a recent visit. Your choice of words and tone of voice can make the process less cumbersome. The following statement is an example of a positive directive: "Mr. Timmons, I know you were just in last week, but I just need to make certain that nothing has changed since your last visit, such as your insurance information, telephone number, etc."

ELIGIBILITY CHECKS

Learning Objective 5: View and perform eligibility checks.

Activity 3-7
View and Perform Eligibility Check—Electronic Eligibility Checks

The *Eligibility* application enables you to view a history of eligibility checks. It also enables you to electronically check eligibility with the primary insurance as well as the secondary insurance saved in *Patient Demographics*. Harris CareTracker PM and EMR automatically performs eligibility checks every evening for all patients scheduled for appointments for the next five days. Automated batch eligibility checks are performed for a patient once every 30 days regardless of the number of appointments scheduled for the patient during that month. However, it is sometimes necessary to perform individual eligibility checks periodically throughout the treatment and payment cycle or for any walk-in patients. The eligibility check helps to identify potential payer sources, reducing the number of denied claims or bad debt write-offs, and decrease staff hours required for performing manual eligibility checks.

Your student version of Harris CareTracker PM does not have the electronic eligibility feature active. To perform the simulated workflow of an eligibility check, you would click the *Elig* button on the dashboard, and then access the payer website or call the insurance company to verify eligibility when electronic access is not available (**Figure 3-18**).

Courtesy of Harris Care Tracker PM and EMR

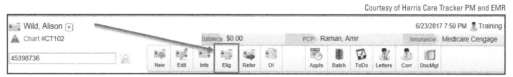

Figure 3-18   Patient Eligibility Button

 SPOTLIGHT   If a patient's primary insurance is a non-participating payer and your practice has not signed up to check eligibility for the payers, the *Elig* button is disabled, preventing you from performing electronic checks. This feature is *not* available on your student version of Harris CareTracker PM.

To perform an eligibility check:

1. Pull patient Alison Wild into context and then click *Elig* on the *Name Bar*. Harris CareTracker PM displays the *Eligibility History* dialog box. In the live version of Harris CareTracker, this box would contain a list of eligibility checks performed for the patient and additional details about the most recent eligibility check. In your student version of Harris CareTracker, you will receive a message stating "No Eligibility History available for this patient."

2. In a live environment, you would click the *Check Eligibility* button in the top right corner to check eligibility. For this activity, you will have to manually simulate checking for patient eligibility. To do this, click the ✎ + *Add Notes* icon to the left of the *Check Eligibility* button. This will open the *Manual Eligibility* box.

3. Enter information into the *Manual Eligibility* box as shown in **Figure 3-19A**.

    a. *Status*: Select "Eligible."

    b. *Verification*: Enter today's date.

    c. *Mark Reviewed*: Select "No."

    d. *Notes*: Enter "Patient is eligible."

    e. Click *Save*.

4. The manual eligibility check will now show in the *Eligibility History* window (**Figure 3-19B**).

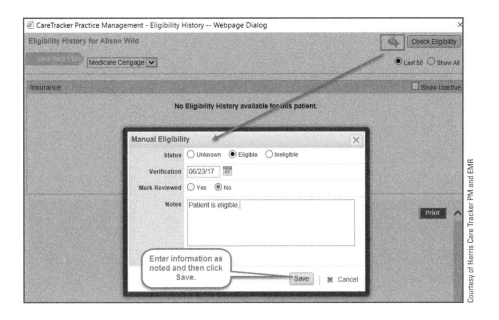

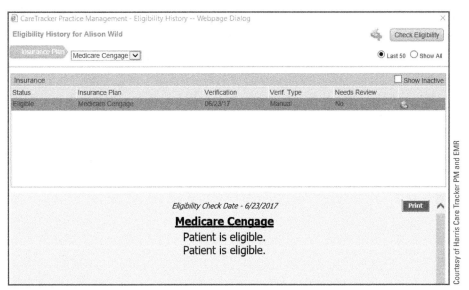

Figures 3-19A and 3-19B   Eligibility Check

 Print the *Eligibility History* screen, label it "Activity 3-7," and place it in your assignment folder.

5. Click "X" in the upper-right corner to close out of the *Eligibility History* window.

> **CRITICAL THINKING**   Now that you have completed your Chapter 3 activities, how did the challenge put forth in the Real-World Connection apply to you? Did you read each activity in its entirety before you started to enter data? Were you accurate in your entries? Did you struggle with any of the activities or steps? If so, which ones? What measures did you take to correct any errors and move forward with the activity, if any?

CASE STUDIES

Case Study 3-1

Repeat Activity 3-1 (Searching for a Patient by Name) for each of the following patients:

a. Alec Winfrey

b. Jim Mcginness

c. Harriet Oshea

Case Study 3-2

Repeat Activity 3-5 (Edit Patient Demographics) and update PCP to the same as the *Group Provider* noted for each of the following patients. Assume that an NPP form has been signed and that requisite consent has been given by each patient and note "Yes" in those fields.

a. Alec Winfrey

b. Jim Mcginness

c. Harriet Oshea

Case Study 3-3

Repeat Activity 3-6 (Print the *Patient Demographics*) for each of the following patients:

a. Alec Winfrey

b. Jim Mcginness

c. Harriet Oshea

Print the Patient Demographics reports, label them "Case Study 3-3A," "Case Study 3-3B," and "Case Study 3-3C," and place them in your assignment folder.

Appointment Scheduling

4

Learning Objectives

1. Book appointments.
2. Check in patients.
3. Set operator preferences, create a batch, accept payments, print patient receipts, run a journal, and post the batch.

Real-World Connection

Answering the phones and scheduling appointments are two of the most challenging tasks in the medical office. These tasks require an individual who is highly organized, can multitask, and has great communication skills. How you communicate with patients is critical to the practice. Not only are you gathering information concerning a patient's health, you must gather accurate information regarding the patient's insurance so that billing the visit is seamless, and revenue is collected in an expedient manner.

Imagine holding the key to your provider's home and controlling which guests have the authority to enter the home and at what times. In some respects, this is similar to what you do when scheduling appointments. Instead of holding the key to the provider's house, you hold the key to the provider's workplace. However, this is only half of the scenario; you must also be cognizant of the severity of the patient's symptoms, the time constraints that prevent the patient from taking the "next available" appointment, and that you have obtained the necessary information for billing.

Consider the desired characteristics of a scheduler as you practice scheduling patients using Harris Care-Tracker PM and think of ways this task impacts billing and coding. The first step to being a good scheduler is becoming familiar with the software! At the end of the chapter, you will be asked to evaluate your experience scheduling patients. Let's begin!

Before you begin the activities in this chapter, refresh your memory on working with Harris CareTracker by referring back to the Best Practices list on page xiv of this workbook. Following best practices will help you complete work quickly and accurately.

BOOK APPOINTMENTS

Learning Objective 1: Book appointments.

Building upon activities in Chapter 3, you will now learn how to book (schedule) appointments.

Activity 4-1
Book an Appointment

Booking appointments in Harris CareTracker PM and EMR takes place in the *Book* application of the *Scheduling* module. Both patient and non-patient appointments (e.g., meetings) are booked in this application. You must have a patient in context in the *Name Bar* to book a patient appointment. Three methods are used to book appointments (**Figure 4-1**):

- Scheduling directly in *Book*: This allows you to book patient and non-patient appointments by manually moving the schedule to a specific day and clicking on a specific time. You can use the *Book* filters to view the schedule for a specific time, day, location, and provider. Scheduling appointments directly from *Book* gives you the advantage of seeing appointment times that can be double-booked.

- Using *Find*: This allows you to search for the next available appointment time based on specific appointment criteria you set. When searching appointment availability, you can filter your search by provider, location, appointment type, date, day, and time.

- Using *Force*: This allows you to double-book appointments and to book an appointment during a different appointment-type time slot. Forced appointments appear outlined in blue on the schedule.

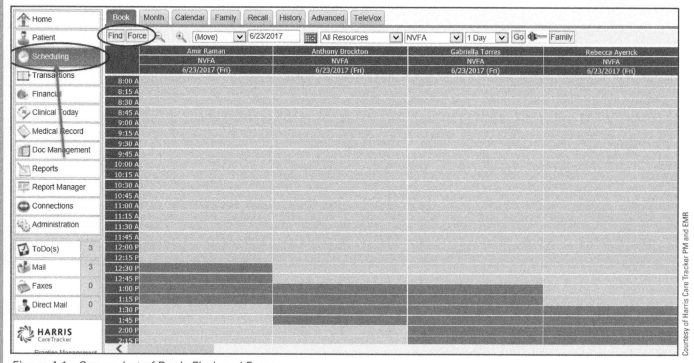

Figure 4-1   Screenshot of Book, Find, and Force

> **ALERT!** You will need to schedule appointments for Activity 4-1 today, or on the next available day this week. Avoid booking appointments too far in advance because it would affect future patient visits and billing activities.

Table 4-1 Patient Appointments to Be Scheduled

PATIENT NAME *PROVIDER*	COMPLAINT	TYPE OF APPOINTMENT: RECORD DATE/TIME SELECTED
Alison Wild *Dr. Raman*	Urinary symptoms	1st available today or this week/Est. Pt. Sick Date: _____ Time: _____
Alec Winfrey *Dr. Raman*	Productive cough; shortness of breath	1st available today or this week/Est. Pt. Sick Date: _____ Time: _____
Jim Mcginness *Dr. Raman*	Back pain, 6 weeks, discuss possible MRI and referral to orthopedist	1st available today or this week/Est. Pt. Sick Date: _____ Time: _____

To Book an Appointment:

Using the instructions below and the patient data in **Table 4-1**, schedule an appointment for each patient on today's date or the next available date this week.

1. Pull the patient for whom you are booking an appointment into context on the *Name Bar*.

2. Click the *Scheduling* module. Harris CareTracker PM and EMR opens the *Book* application by default.

3. Display the desired date using one of the following options:

   a. Select an option from the *Move* list to display the schedule for specific time increments such as Next Day, Next Week, 2 Months, and so on.

   b. Manually enter a date in MM/DD/YYYY format or click the *Calendar* icon to display the schedule for a specific date.

4. Select the provider, location, and the number of days to display, and then click *Go* (**Figure 4-2**).

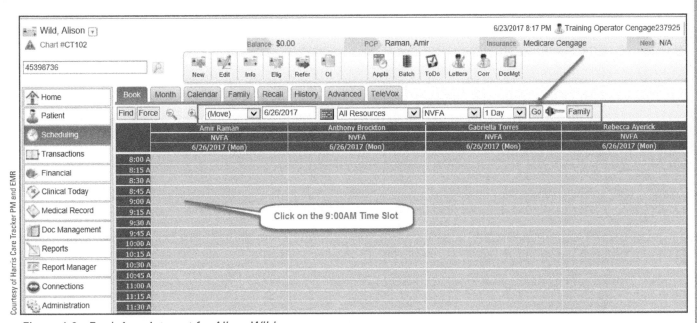

Figure 4-2 Book Appointment for Alison Wild

5. Click on the time slot for which you are booking the appointment with Dr. Amir Raman. (If the schedule is displayed for multiple providers and locations, be sure to click the time slot in the appropriate column.) The application displays the *Book Appointment* window.

 TIP If the patient has existing appointments scheduled, the application displays the *Existing Appointments* window. Click *Book Appointment* at the bottom of the window to book a new appointment.

6. From the *Appointment Type* list, select the appointment type. When you select an appointment type, Harris CareTracker PM and EMR automatically populates the *Task* and *Duration* fields (**Figure 4-3**).

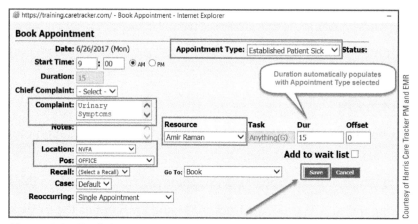

Figure 4-3   Book Appointment Window for Alison Wild

7. From the *Resource* list, select the resource (i.e., provider) needed for the appointment (select Amir Raman, if not already populated).

8. There are two options for entering a *Chief Complaint* (you can only use option [a]):

   a. Free text the chief complaint (as noted in Table 4-1) in the *Complaint* box (see Figure 4-3). For example, enter "Urinary Symptoms" for patient Alison Wild. (The application will display the complaint in brackets [ ] next to the patient's name on the schedule.)

   b. (FYI) From the *Chief Complaint* list, select a chief complaint from the drop-down list. This list is populated with the favorite complaints selected in the *Chief Complaint Maintenance* application in the *Administration* module. (This is not available in your student version. You will use the "free text" option.)

9. In the *Notes* box, enter any notes about the appointment (there are no notes associated with the patients in Table 4-1). (Notes appear in parentheses next to the patient's name on the schedule and also appear when you move your mouse over the appointment on the schedule.)

 TIP Do not use any symbols when entering appointment notes or patient complaints. Using symbols will cause an error when you try to print encounter forms.

10. From the *Location* list, select "NVFA."

11. From the *Pos* (Place of Service) list, select "OFFICE."

12. Do not link the appointment to an open recall for the patient.

13. Do not link the patient's appointment to a specific case.

14. Do not select recurring appointment.

15. Click *Save*. The application schedules the appointment. Now repeat steps 1 through 15 for patients Alec Winfrey and Jim Mcginness (**Figure 4-4**).

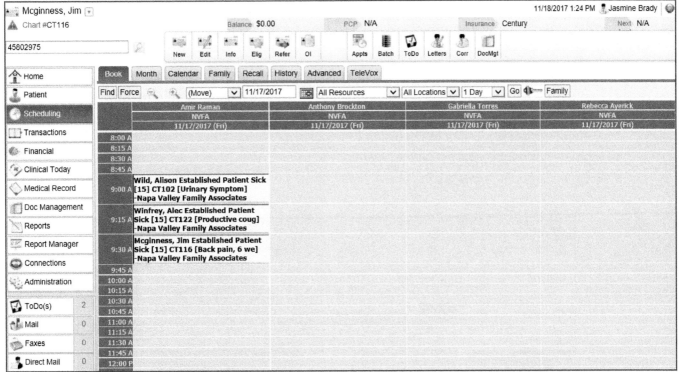

Figure 4-4   Scheduled Appointment for Alison Wild

Courtesy of Harris Care Tracker PM and EMR

 Print a screenshot of the Schedule/Booking screen with each patient scheduled (from Table 4-1), label it "Activity 4-1," and place it in your assignment folder.

PROFESSIONALISM CONNECTION

At times it may be necessary to double-book appointments. This often occurs during flu season, or when a patient is acutely ill and needs to be seen the day of the appointment request. When this is the case, always check with the provider first. Make certain that the provider is on board with being double-booked. If you are unable to accommodate the patient, weigh all other options before discontinuing the call. Check to see if any other providers are available to see the patient, or when possible, refer the patient to an urgent care facility connected with your organization. Always demonstrate a caring attitude toward the patient, and when unable to accommodate the patient's specific preferences, offer an apology while you work to explore additional options for the patient.

CHECK IN PATIENTS

Learning Objective 2: Check in patients.

Activity 4-2

Check In Patient from the Mini-Menu

For a patient encounter to be generated in the electronic medical record (EMR), the patient must be checked in when he or she arrives for an appointment. Checking in a patient changes his or her Harris CareTracker PM and EMR status to "Checked In," and verifies that the patient's billing and demographic information is complete. Harris CareTracker PM and EMR will display the *Patient Alert* dialog box if the patient is missing important billing or demographic data.

 TIP *Patient Alerts* will only display if the *Show Alerts* feature is activated in your batch.

You can check in a patient in Harris CareTracker PM and EMR in the following places:

- In the *Book* application of the *Scheduling* module, using the mini-menu drop-down feature (**Figure 4-5**).
- From the *Appts* button in the *Name Bar*.
- From the *Appointments list* on the *Dashboard*.
- From the *Appointments* tab in *Clinical Today*.

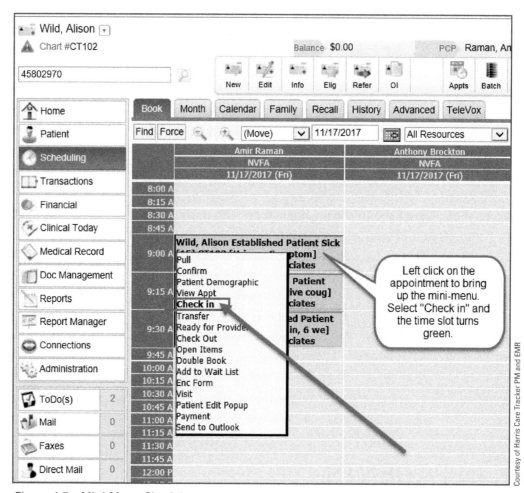

Figure 4-5   Mini-Menu Check-In

Check In Patient from Mini Menu:

1. You will check in the following patients in this activity:

   a. Alison Wild

   b. Alec Winfrey

   c. Jim Mcginness

Before you begin this activity, refer back to the dates of the appointments you scheduled for each of them in Activity 4-1. If you did not record their appointment dates, pull the patient into context, click on the *Scheduling* module, and click on the *History* tab. All of the patient's appointments will be displayed. Once you have the patients' appointment dates in hand, continue to step 2.

2. Click the *Scheduling* module. Harris CareTracker PM opens the *Book* application by default.

3. With or without the patient in context, move the schedule to display the appointment for the patient you want to check in. This can be done by manually entering in the date in the *Date* box, by clicking the *Calendar* ⊞ icon, or by selecting a time period from the *Move* list. Be sure that "All Resources" and "All Locations" display. If not, use the drop-down, change the parameters, and click *Go*.

4. Left-click the name of the patient you want to check in and select *Check in* from the mini-menu (see Figure 4-5). Harris CareTracker PM changes the patient's status to "Checked In" and highlights the patient's appointment in green in both the *Book* application and the *Appointments* link in the *Front Office* section of the *Dashboard* (*Home* module). Checking in a patient from the mini-menu will pull the patient into context. **FYI:** Harris CareTracker PM and EMR records the check-in time and displays the patient's wait time in the *Appointments* link (**Figure 4-6**). For all the patients to appear in the *Appointments* link, be sure to change the *Resource* to *All*, enter the date you want to check status for, and select *All* from the *Status* drop-down.

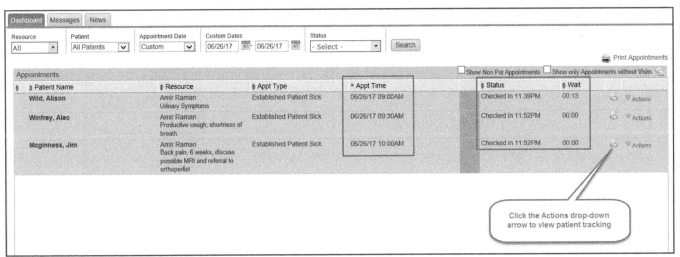

Figure 4-6   Check-In Wait Time

Courtesy of Harris Care Tracker PM and EMR

5. Repeat steps 2 through 4 until you have all patients from step 1 checked in.

🖨 **Print a screenshot of the Schedule screen with the patient checked in, label it "Activity 4-2," and place it in your assignment folder.**

CREATE A BATCH

Learning Objective 3: Set Operator preferences, create a batch, accept payments, print patient receipts, run a journal, and post the batch.

Activity 4-3
Setting Operator Preferences

The *Batch* application is used for setting defaults for both "Financial" and "Clinical" components. The "Financial" portion of the batch establishes defaults and assigns a name to a batch (group) of financial transactions you will be entering into Harris CareTracker PM and EMR. A new financial batch is created daily to enter financial transactions into Harris CareTracker PM and EMR, for example, charges, payments, and adjustments. This helps identify transactions linked to the batch, the date of each transaction, and the operator who entered it into the system. Setting up the financial batch helps identify a group of charges or payments and helps run reports to balance against the actual charges or payments entered.

The "Clinical" batch settings are typically set up only once and are used to set preferences and pre-populate fields common to your workflow (**Figure 4-7**). The "Clinical" batch settings are in the middle and lower sections of the *Operator Encounter Batch Control* dialog box. Setting the defaults here can speed up scheduling by having default *Resource* and *Location* defined.

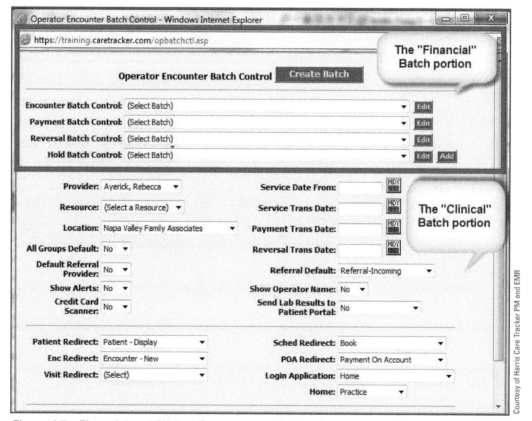

Figure 4-7   Financial and Clinical Components of a Batch

Courtesy of Harris Care Tracker PM and EMR

Setting Operator Preferences

The *Batch* application enables you to set up operator preferences based on the workflow for your role. This reduces the number of clicks required to get from one application to the other, making navigation through Harris CareTracker PM and EMR easy.

The first time you log in to Harris CareTracker you will be prompted to create a batch. Activities related to searching for a patient or scheduling a patient do not require that a batch be created. For the activities related to financial and clinical, you will need to have a batch open. You begin by setting your operator preferences.

The available batch redirects are described in **Table 4-2**. These are located in the lower section of the *Operator Encounter Batch Control* dialog box (**Figure 4-8**).

Table 4-2   Batch Redirects

REDIRECTS *FIELD*	DESCRIPTION
Patient Redirect	Launches the selected application after editing a *Demographic* record in the *Patient* module. You can also change this setting in the *Demographic* application if necessary.
Enc Redirect	Launches the selected application after saving a *Charge* in the *Transactions* module.
Visit Redirect	Launches the selected application after a visit is saved in the *Visit* application.
Sched Redirect	Launches the selected application after an appointment is booked via the *Book* application of the *Scheduling* module.
POA (Payment on Account) Redirect	Launches the selected application after a payment is entered via the *Payment on Account* application of the *Transaction* module.
Login Application	Launches the selected application when you log in to Harris CareTracker PM and EMR.
Home	If the *Log in Application* is set to "Home," you can select which *Home* module application to display by default. For example, the *Management, Meaningful Use, Messages*, or *News* applications.
When finished with redirects, click *Save*	Your screen will be saved with selections made.

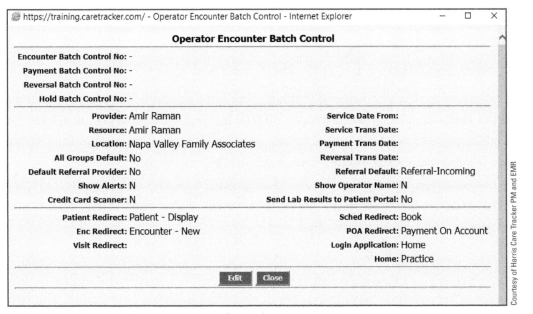

Figure 4-8   Operator Encounter Batch Control

To Set Operator Preferences:

1. With no patient in context, click *Batch* ▌ on the *Name Bar*. Harris CareTracker PM and EMR displays the *Operator Encounter Batch Control* dialog box.

2. If there is an open batch, by default the batch will display. Harris CareTracker PM and EMR assigns redirects, making it easy to navigate from different applications within Harris CareTracker PM and EMR. The default redirects are based on the most commonly used workflow. Redirect means to change the path or direction; for example, changing a redirect allows the operator to select the most efficient workflow.

3. Click *Edit* if the fields are grayed out. Otherwise, enter (or confirm if already populated) the information for each of the fields in the *Operator Encounter Batch Control* dialog box (see Figure 4-8) as follows:

   a. Patient Redirect: (Select "Patient – Display")

   b. Enc Redirect: (Select "Encounter – New")

   c. Visit Redirect: (Select "Select")

   d. Sched Redirect: (Select "Book")

   e. POA (Payment on Account) Redirect: (Select "Payment on Account")

   f. Login Application: (Select "Home")

   g. Home: (Select "Practice")

4. Click *Save*. Screen will be saved with selections made.

5. Click *Close* to close out the batch control box.

📇 **Print a screenshot of the Operator Encounter Batch Control screen, label it "Activity 4-3," and place it in your assignment folder.**

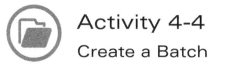

Activity 4-4
Create a Batch

A provider's paperless desk is incorporated in the *Clinical Today* module. Therefore, selecting the *Clinical* module from the *Login Application* list takes you directly to the *Clinical Today* module each time you log in to Harris CareTracker PM and EMR, streamlining workflow. When you begin clinical activities in Chapter 6, you will change your *Login Application* to the *Clinical* setting.

Having set up your operator preferences in the *Operator Encounter Batch Control* in Activity 4-3 and with the dialog box in display, you will now create a batch. Reference the instructions and fields in **Table 4-3** as you complete your batch details.

Table 4-3 Batch Details Field and Instructions

FIELD	INSTRUCTIONS
Provider	From the *Provider* list, select the name of the billing provider associated with the batch. **Note:** The *Admissions* application accessed via the *Dashboard* and the *Charges* application in the *Transactions* module displays the billing provider set up in the batch.
Resource	From the *Resource* list, select the servicing provider. In most instances, the billing provider and the resource are the same. **Note:** The *Book* application in the *Scheduling* module and the *Appointment* application in the *Clinical Today* module display the resource set up in the batch.
Location	From the *Location* list, select the location associated with the batch. **Note:** The *Admissions* application accessed via the *Dashboard* and the *Book* application in the *Scheduling* module displays the location set up in the batch.
All Groups Default	By default, the *All Groups Default* list is set to "No." Change the list to "Yes" if necessary. This displays patient financial information for the current group or all groups in the practice based on the setting selected. If "Yes" is selected, you can only see the financial transactions for the groups that you have access to as an operator. This setting mostly benefits multi-group practices and also determines the default value in the *Open Items* application of the *Financial* module and *Edit* application of the *Transactions* module.
Default Referral Provider	By default, the *Default Referral Provider* list is set to "No." Change the field to "Yes" if there is no referring provider in the patient's demographics or if there is no active referral/authorization for the patient. This sets the billing provider as the referring provider.
Show Alerts	In the *Show Alerts* field, select "Yes" to enable Harris CareTracker PM to display the *Patient Alert* window; otherwise select "No." The *Patient Alerts* window notifies users when key information is missing from a patient's demographics or when there are other issues with a patient's account.
Credit Card Scanner	The *Credit Card Scanner* field is set to *"No"* by default. Your student version of Harris CareTracker will NOT have this feature. In a real practice setting, select *"Yes"* if your group uses a credit card scanner to process payments by credit card.
Service Date From	Click the *Calendar* icon and select the start of the service dates included in the batch.
Service Trans Date	Click the *Calendar* icon and select the service transaction date included in the batch.
Payment Trans Date	Click the *Calendar* icon and select the payment transactions date included in the batch.
Reversal Trans Date	Click the *Calendar* icon and select the reversal transactions date included in the batch.
Referral Default	By default, the *Referral Default* list is set to "Referral-Incoming." Select a referral type based on your practice specialty. The selected option will display as the default option when the *Ref/Auth* application is accessed via the *Name Bar* or *Patient* module.
Show Operator Name	Select "Yes" to display the operator's name on the Harris CareTracker PM and EMR interface. Select "No" if you do not want the operator's name displayed.
Click *Save*. The batch information is saved.	
Note: Click *Edit* to make changes if necessary.	
Click "X" on the right-hand corner to close the dialog box.	

To Create a Batch:

1. Before creating a batch, make sure your fiscal period and fiscal year are open for the month(s) in which patient appointments are scheduled (refer to Activities 2-4 and 2-5 if you need to refresh your memory). For example, if Alison Wild's appointment is in June 2017, make sure the fiscal period June 2017 is open. Once you have confirmed the fiscal period and year are open, proceed to step 2. **Note**: If you are working at the month's end and are booking appointments in the following month, you would need to open the current <u>and</u> next month in fiscal period. This would also apply to the fiscal period selected in your batch.

2. Click on the *Batch* icon on the *Name Bar*. Then click *Edit*, and then click *Create Batch*. The *Batch Master* dialog box displays (**Figure 4-9**).

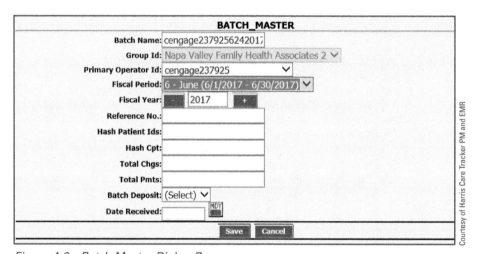

Figure 4-9   Batch Master Dialog Box

3. By default, the *Batch Name* field displays a batch identification name. The name consists of your user-name followed by the current date. (**Note:** You can edit the batch name if necessary to identify the types of financial transactions associated with the batch; for example, "copayment5132017.") Do not use symbols when editing the name. Change the Batch Name to "FrontOfficeCopayment" (**Figure 4-10**).

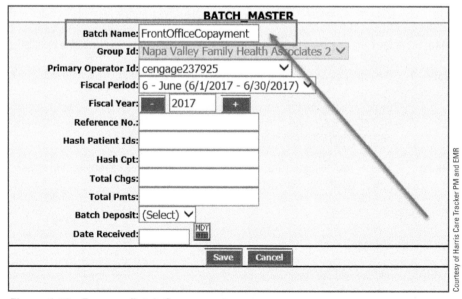

Figure 4-10   Rename Batch Copayment

4. By default, the *Group Id* displays the name of your group.

5. By default, the *Primary Operator Id* displays your username.

6. In the *Fiscal Period* field, click the month in which patients from Activity 4-1 have appointments. The list will only display fiscal periods that are currently open.

7. By default, the *Fiscal Year* displays the current financial year set up for your company in Activity 2-4.

8. *Hash Patient Ids* box—Leave blank for this activity. **(FYI)** The *Hash Patient Ids* box is where the person entering the batch data would enter the sum of all patient Harris CareTracker PM and EMR ID numbers pertaining to the charges associated with the batch. This is to ensure that a charge is entered for all patients associated with the batch.

9. *Hash Cpt* box—Leave blank for this activity. **(FYI)** The *Hash Cpt* box is where you enter the sum of all CPT® codes pertaining to the charges associated with the batch. This is to ensure that a charge is entered for all procedures. Example: If two patients are seen for the day, and the CPT® codes selected on the encounter form for the first patient are 71101 and 99213, and the second patient are 71101 and 99203, calculate the *Hash CPT* by adding 71101 + 99213 + 71101 + 99203 = 340618.

10. *Total Chgs* box—Leave blank for this activity. **(FYI)** The *Total Chgs* box is where you enter the sum of all charges that are associated with the batch.

11. *Total Pmts* box—Leave blank for this activity. **(FYI)** The *Total Pmts* box is where you enter the sum of check(s) that are associated with the batch.

12. *Batch Deposit* list—Leave blank for this activity. **(FYI)** The *Batch Deposit* list is where you would select the *Deposit ID* to link to a deposit number, if using the *Batch Deposit* application. (This feature is not active in your student version.)

13. *Date Received* box—Leave blank for this activity. **(FYI)** You could enter the date the encounter was received in MM/DD/YYYY format or click the *Calendar* icon and select the date.

14. Click *Save*. You may receive a message box asking if you are sure you want to select the fiscal period. After confirming the correct fiscal period is displaying, click *OK*. Harris CareTracker PM and EMR displays the *Operator Encounter Batch Control* dialog box with the new batch information (**Figure 4-11**).

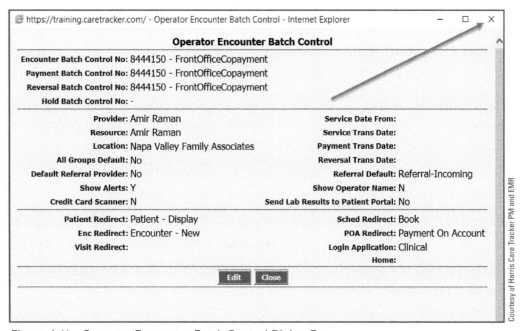

Figure 4-11   Operator Encounter Batch Control Dialog Box

15. Now, further edit your batch by updating the provider, resource, location, and so on (the middle section of the *Operator Encounter Batch Control* box). Select the *Provider* (Amir Raman), *Resource* (Amir Raman), and *Location* (Napa Valley Family Associates).

16. Click *Save*.

17. Write down your "Encounter Batch Control No." for future reference. (Should include "Copayment") _____ .

🖳 **Print a screenshot of the Batch screen, label it "Activity 4-4," and place it in your assignment folder.**

18. Click "*X*" in the top right-hand corner to close the *Batch* dialog box.

Activity 4-5
Accept/Enter a Payment

The *Payments On Account (Pmt on Acc)* application is used to record patient payments. Typically, you will accept a patient's copayment at the check-in process. A copayment is a predetermined (flat) fee that an individual pays for health care services in addition to what the insurance covers. For example, some health maintenance organizations (HMOs) require a $25 "copayment" for each office visit, regardless of the type or level of services provided during the visit. Copayments are not usually specified by percentages. You can access the *Payments on Account* application from the following locations within practice management:

- *Scheduling* module > *Book* tab > left-click on the patient's appointment in the schedule to display the Mini-Menu > Select *Payment* link
- *Name Bar* > *Appts* button > *Actions* menu *Payment* link
- *Transactions* module > *Pmt on Acct* tab
- *Transactions* module > *Charge* tab

To Accept/Enter a Payment:

1. Pull patient Alec Winfrey into context.

2. In the *Transactions* module, click on the *Pmt on Acct* tab.

3. From the drop-down list at the top of the screen, select whether the payment is being made by the *Patient* or *Responsible Party*. (Select "Patient.")

4. If a patient is paying a portion of his or her balance (or copayment), enter the dollar amount of the payment in the *Amount* box. (Enter "$35.00.")

   (FYI) If the patient is paying his or her entire balance (or copayment), click *Pay Bal*. Harris CareTracker PM and EMR automatically pulls the patient's balance into the *Amount* box.

5. From the *Payment Type* list, select the payment method. (Select "Payment – Patient Check.")
   (**Note:** If the payment type is credit card, you would select the *Process Credit Card* checkbox.)

6. If the payment method is a check, enter the check number in the *Reference #* box (enter "2014" as the check number). The reference number will print on the patient's receipt.

7. From the *Method* list, select how to apply the payment to the patient's account:

    a. If you are collecting a copayment for a patient who does not have an outstanding balance, select <u>only</u> "Force Unapplied." Harris CareTracker PM and EMR creates an unapplied balance for the patient that is applied to the patient's private pay balance when his or her charges are saved.

    b. Because Mr. Winfrey has a scheduled appointment, select "Force Unapplied" and check the *Copay?* box.

    (FYI): If the patient has an outstanding balance you would:

- Select *Today's First* in the *Method* field to apply the money starting with the most current balance and then back toward the oldest date of service for which the patient has an outstanding balance.

- Select *Oldest to Newest* in the *Method* field to apply the money to the oldest date of service for which the patient has an outstanding balance and then forward toward the most current date of service.

8. In the *Trans. Date* box, enter the transaction date to which you want to link the payment. Because you are entering a copayment for a patient visit, select the date of the patient's appointment you scheduled in Activity 4-1. **Note**: If you had selected dates in your batch defaults when you set up your batch, they would prepopulate. **Hint**: If you are working at the month's end and are booking appointments in the following month, you would need to open both the current and next month in fiscal period. This would also apply to the fiscal period selected in your batch.

    (FYI): The following are the various Transaction Date Defaults:

- If a transaction date was selected when you created your batch, Harris CareTracker PM and EMR pulls that date into the *Trans. Date* box.

- If a transaction date was not selected, the transaction date defaults to the date in your batch name.

- If there is no date in your batch name, the transaction date defaults to the date the payment is entered in Harris CareTracker PM and EMR.

9. Because this is a copay:

    a. Select the *Copay?* checkbox.

    b. In the *Appt* field, select the appointment date to which the copay applies (the appointment scheduled in Activity 4-1), if possible. (**Note:** You cannot link a copay to a future appointment date. If your appointment is in the future, you won't be able to select it, and you can skip this step.)

    c. **FYI:** The *Plan Name* and *Copay Amt* fields display the insurance plan and copay amount saved in the patient's demographics, if applicable. These fields are read-only.

 TIP The *Plan Name* and *Copay Amt* fields display the insurance plan and copay amount saved in the patient's demographics, if applicable. These fields are read-only.

10. The *Go To* field defaults to the redirect option selected in the operator's batch. You can select a different option if needed (**Figure 4-12**). (Select "Payment on Account.")

11. To view a summary of the transaction prior to saving, click *View Trans* (**Figure 4-13**). **Note**: If you do not need to view the transaction, you can click directly on *Quick Save* to save the transaction.

12. After clicking *View Trans*, click *Save*. Harris CareTracker PM and EMR saves the payment information and launches the application selected in the *Go To* field. (You selected the *Go To* of *Payment on Account* that brings you back to the original *Pmt on Acct* tab.)

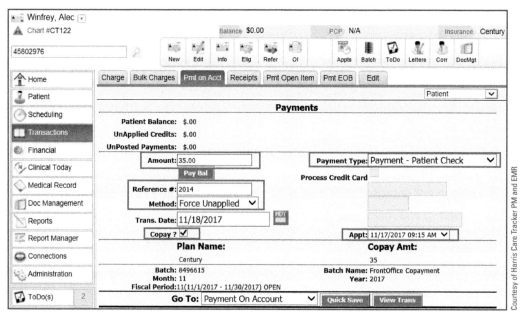

Figure 4-12 Enter Payment on Account

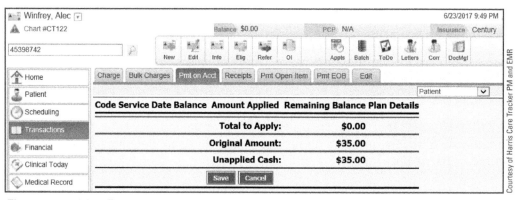

Figure 4-13 View Transaction

ALERT! Do *NOT* post the batch.

13. Click on the *Home* module and the *Open Batches* link under the *Billing* header on the *Dashboard* (**Figure 4-14**) to view your batch with the payment recorded. **Note:** Only view the batch, do not post it.

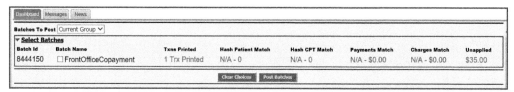

Figure 4-14 Open Batches

Courtesy of Harris Care Tracker PM and EMR

14. You will later print a receipt from the *Receipts* tab in the *Transactions* module (Activity 4-6).

📠 **Print the Open Batch screen, label it "Activity 4-5," and place it in your assignment folder.**

PROFESSIONALISM CONNECTION

Some patients feel that medicine and money should never mix; however, a medical office is a business and must conduct itself as such. This means that collecting the copayment prior to the visit makes the most business sense. Once the appointment is completed, the services have been rendered and the patient may not be as willing to meet his or her financial obligations. When possible, the collection of payments should be performed outside of the reception area; however, when this is not possible, the collection of payments should be handled in a discreet manner. You may use a phrase such as the following: "Mrs. Barrett, what method of payment will you be using today to meet your copayment requirement?" This sentence illustrates that payment is expected, but you are willing to work with the patient by accepting a mode of payment that works best for her.

Activity 4-6

Print Patient Receipts

After entering the payment information in Activity 4-5, print a receipt from the *Receipts* tab in the *Transactions* module. Receipts in Harris CareTracker PM and EMR identify a patient's previous balance, the activity of charges and payments for that date of service, and the new patient balance.

1. With the patient in context (Alec Winfrey), click the *Transactions* module. **Note:** You will still be working in the *Batch* you created in Activity 4-3. **Hint:** If you are working at the month's end and are booking appointments in the following month, you would need to open the current <u>and</u> next month in fiscal period. This would also apply to the fiscal period selected in your batch.

2. When the *Transactions* module opens, click on the *Receipts* tab.

3. From the drop-down list at the top of the screen, select who you would like to view the receipt from, *Patient* or *Responsible Party*. (Select "Patient.")

4. Select the date of service for which you need to print a receipt from the *Receipts* list. (Select the date of the payment received, which should also be the same date as your batch and the date that matches the patient's appointment.) When a date of service is selected, the receipt displays on the screen.

5. Click on the *Print* button (**Figure 4-15**), or right-click on the receipt. When you right-click, a gray pop-up menu appears. Select *Print*, and the receipt will print.

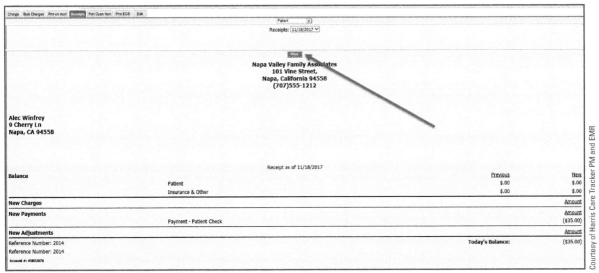

Figure 4-15   Print Patient Receipt

Print the Patient Receipt, label it "Activity 4-6," and place it in your assignment folder.

Activity 4-7

Accept/Enter a Payment and Print a Receipt

1. Repeat Activity 4-5 for patient Jim Mcginness and accept/enter a copay for his appointment you scheduled in Activity 4-1:

   a. Amount $35.00

   b. Paid by check #5513

2. Click back on the *Receipts* tab and print the *Receipt*.

 Print the Patient Receipt, label it "Activity 4-7", and place it in your assignment folder.

 PROFESSIONALISM CONNECTION

In a hurry, the check-in desk did not confirm Jim's demographic information or scan a copy of his current insurance card. Jim's employer changed to a new health insurance plan, Blue Shield Cengage (ID #BCBS987) on the first day of last month. His new copay is $20.00. Keep this in mind and think about how the erroneous copayment will affect the billing function in later activities.

Activity 4-8

Run a Journal

Now that you have entered copayments, you will complete the process by running a journal and posting your batch as your "end-of-day" workflow.

You must run a journal prior to posting your batch (Activity 4-9) to verify that you have entered all the financial transactions correctly in Harris CareTracker PM and EMR. Journals provide a summary of financial transactions, for example, charges, payments, and adjustments.

It is important to identify and correct any errors before a batch is posted. Once a batch has been posted, the transactions linked to it are locked in the system and must be reversed to be corrected. Posted errors can only be corrected by reversing the transaction on the patient's account, which occurs in the *Edit* application of the *Transactions* module. It is highly recommended that you run a journal before posting your batch to make sure that your transactions for the day are correct and balance.

Posted batches are accessible any time so you can always access an old journal from the *Historical Journals* link (**Figure 4-16**) under the *Financial Reports* section of the *Reports* application, which alleviates the need to save paper copies of journals.

To Run a Journal:

1. Click the *Reports* module.

2. Click the *Todays Journals* link under the *Financial Reports* section (**Figure 4-17**). Harris CareTracker displays the *Todays Journal Options* screen (see **Figure 4-18**). All of your group's open batches are listed in the *Todays Batches* box.

3. Select a batch to include in the journal either by double-clicking on the batch name or by clicking on the batch and then clicking *Add* (**Figure 4-19**). Harris CareTracker PM and EMR adds the selected batches to the box on the right. (Add batch "FrontOfficeCopayment.")

4. From the *Sort By* list drop-down, select "Entry Date."

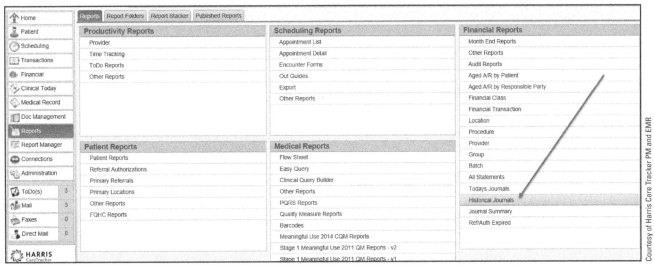

Figure 4-16   Historical Journals Link

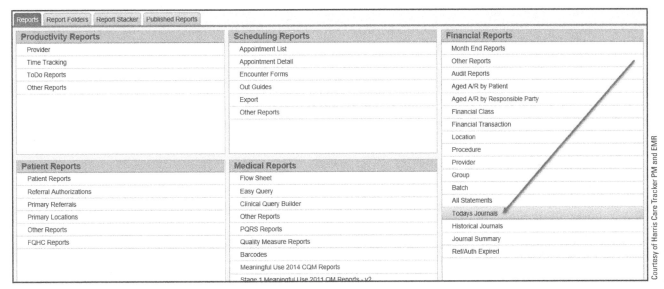

Figure 4-17   Todays Journals Link

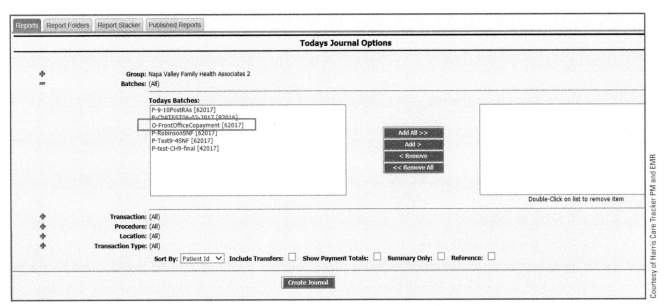

Figure 4-18   Todays Journal Options

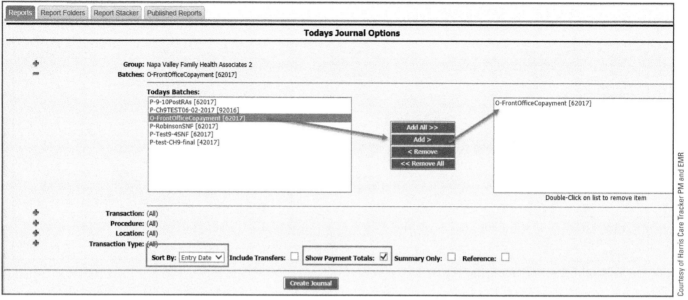

Figure 4-19   Select a Batch for the Journal

5. Select the *Show Payment Totals* checkbox (see Figure 4-19).

6. Click *Create Journal*. Harris CareTracker PM generates the journal (**Figure 4-20**).

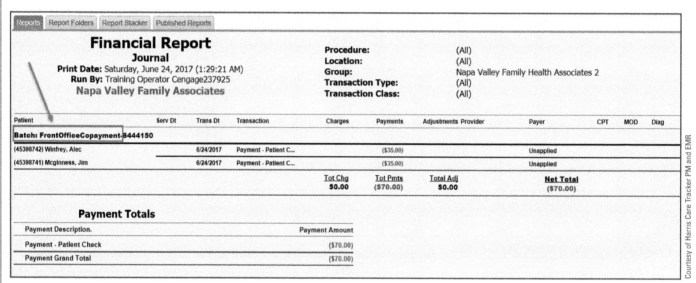

Figure 4-20   Journal

7. To print, right-click on the journal and select *Print* from the shortcut menu.

🖳 **Print the Journal screen, label it "Activity 4-8," and place it in your assignment folder.**

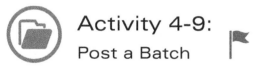

Activity 4-9:
Post a Batch

After reviewing the transactions in your journal for accuracy, you will post your open batch. Batches should only be posted after a journal has been generated and you have verified your journal balances. Posting batches locks the transactions permanently in Harris CareTracker. All transactions will show on reports generated in Harris CareTracker, and any corrections to posted transactions must be made via the

Edit application in the *Transactions* module. *Open Batches* can also be viewed and posted by clicking on the *Open Batches* link under the *Billing* section of the *Dashboard* on the *Home* page. After generating a journal for the batch(es), you would like to post, review, identify, and correct transactions errors, if any, prior to posting the batch.

To Post Your Batch:

1. Click the *Administration* module. The application opens the *Practice* tab.

2. Click the *Post* link under the *Daily Administration > Financial* header (**Figure 4-21**). Harris CareTracker PM displays a list of all open batches for the group.

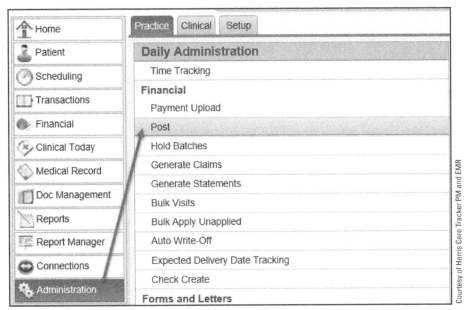

Figure 4-21   Post Link from Admin Practice Tab

3. Select the checkbox next to the batch you want to post. (Select batch "FrontOfficeCopayment.")

🖬 **Print the Post Batch screen, label it "Activity 4-9," and place it in your assignment folder.**

4. Click *Post Batches* (**Figure 4-22**).

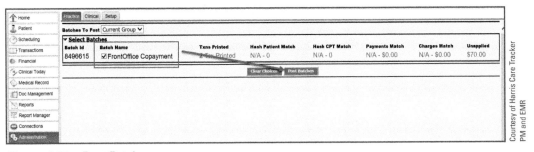

Figure 4-22   Post Batches

An alternative way of posting batches is via the *Open Batches* link on the Home > *Dashboard*, under the *Billing* header. Although not required, it is recommended to only post a batch after a journal has been generated and balances verified. The total number of open batches for your group displays next to the *Open Batches* link.

CRITICAL THINKING   Now that you have completed this chapter's activities, how do you feel about the scheduling and financial responsibilities of a medical assistant? Were you able to follow instructions and accurately schedule patients, receive and post copayments, and create and post a batch? Were there any activities or steps that seemed to be difficult and challenging? If so, which ones? What measures did you take to accurately complete the activities and move forward? What are your impressions of the front office administrative staff that must balance their responsibilities? If you become a front office medical assistant, what skills and key attributes can you comfortably say you can offer to your employer?

CASE STUDY
Case Study 4-1
Repeat Activity 4-6 (Print Patient Receipts) for patient Jim Mcginness.

💾 **Print a receipt for Jim Mcginness, label it "Case Study 4-1," and place it in your assignment folder.**

Preliminary Duties in the EMR and Patient Work-Up

5

Learning Objectives

1. Define meaningful use and list its stages.
2. Describe tools within Harris CareTracker PM and EMR that assist with meaningful use.
3. View the meaningful use dashboard in Harris CareTracker PM and EMR.
4. Activate the care management registries in Harris CareTracker PM and EMR.
5. Set operator preferences in your Batch application.
6. List major applications of the Clinical Today module.
7. View daily appointments in Clinical Today.
8. Perform check-in duties and track patients throughout their visits.
9. Retrieve the patient's EMR and update sections within the patient health history panes.
10. Update the Patient Care Management application.
11. Create and print a Progress Note.

Real-World Connection

In the first four chapters, you learned a great deal about the practice management side of the Harris CareTracker software. This chapter introduces you to the EMR components and focuses on the utilization of EMRs in ambulatory care settings. For providers to obtain full reimbursement from governmental agencies such as Medicare and Medicaid, they must be in full compliance with specific guidelines set forth by those agencies.

EMRs have been in use for the past couple of decades, but their widespread adoption skyrocketed largely due to Medicare and Medicaid financial incentives offered by the federal government for practices that meet meaningful use as well as the penalties that come about for not instituting and meaningfully using the EMR. As you work in this chapter, keep in mind how your position as a medical assistant may be impacted by meaningful use, and how you will be able to assist both providers and patients in meeting these goals.

In this chapter, you are going to learn a great deal about working in the patient's electronic medical record (EMR). You are very fortunate to enter the medical field at a time when technology is flourishing. Electronic medical records organize the patient's information so that you know exactly where each item is stored within the patient's chart. EMRs also help medical assistants stay on task and keep up with lab reports and prescription renewals. Your challenge is to embrace the training in this chapter so that you are able to fully navigate the patient's medical record in Harris CareTracker EMR.

Although this workbook focuses primarily on billing and coding functions, it is important to have an understanding of all administrative and clinical duties a medical assistant may be tasked with. How can you, as a medical coder and biller, be a part of the team that delivers quality patient care?

> Before you begin the activities in this chapter, refresh your memory on working with Harris CareTracker by referring back to the Best Practices list on page xiv of this workbook. Following best practices will help you complete work quickly and accurately.

ELECTRONIC MEDICAL RECORDS

Learning Objective 1: Define meaningful use and list its stages.

Learning Objective 2: Describe tools within Harris CareTracker PM and EMR that assist with meaningful use.

Learning Objective 3: View the meaningful use dashboard in Harris CareTracker PM and EMR.

Learning Objective 4: Activate the care management registries in Harris CareTracker PM and EMR.

Meaningful Use

Meaningful use is the way in which EHR technologies must be implemented and used for a provider to be eligible for the EHR Incentive Programs and to qualify for incentive payments. These incentives specify three components of meaningful use:

- The use of a certified EHR in a meaningful manner
- The use of certified EHR technology for electronic exchange of health information to improve quality of health care
- The use of certified EHR technology to submit clinical quality and other measures

The purpose of meaningful use is to not only institute the adoption of EMRs but also ascertain that practices use their EHR software to its fullest. Benefits of meaningful use include complete and accurate medical records, better access to information, and patient empowerment. One of the major goals of meaningful use is to make medical records interoperable so that immediate access can be given to any provider who works with the patient. Three stages are associated with meaningful use.

Stage 1: Data Capture and Sharing Stage

This stage focuses on the following:

- Electronic capturing of health information in a coded format
- Using electronically captured health information to track key clinical conditions and communicate information for care coordination purposes
- Implementing clinical decision support tools to facilitate disease and medication management
- Reporting information for quality improvement and public health information

Meaningful Use Criteria for Eligible Professionals

Meaningful use criteria require providers to meet 14 core objectives, 5 out of 10 menu set objectives, and 6 total clinical quality measures. **Figures 5-1A** and **5-1B** illustrate what is included in the core and menu set objectives. (In Figure 5-1A, please note that core objective C-12 was required through 2013, but will not be a requirement moving forward.) Stage 1 was implemented in 2011 and 2012.

List of Core Requirements - Final Regulation

ARRA EHR MEANINGFUL USE STAGE 1 REQUIREMENTS

CT #	CORE REQUIREMENTS (must meet all of these)
C 1	Record demographics as structured data for preferred language, race, ethnicity, date of birth, and gender (50 percent requirement).
C 2	Record and chart changes in vital signs (BP, height, weight, & display BMI); additionally, plot and display growth charts for children age 2 to 20 including BMI (50 percent requirement).
C 3	Maintain an up-to-date problem list of current and active diagnoses based on ICD-9-CM or SNOMED CT (80 percent of all unique patients admitted have at least one entry or an indication of "no problems are known" recorded as structured data).
C 4	Maintain active medication list with at least one entry or indication of "no currently prescribed medications" as structured data (80 percent requirement).
C 5	Maintain active medication allergy list with at least one entry or indication of "no known medication allergies" as structured data (80 percent requirement).
C 6	Record smoking status for patients 13 years old or older as structured data (50 percent requirement).
C 7	Provide patient with clinical summary for patients for each office visit within 3 business days (more than 50 percent for all office visits).
C 8	Provide patients with electronic copy of their health information (problems, medication, medication allergies, diagnostic test results) upon request (50 percent of patients must receive electronic copy within three days).
C 9	Generate and transmit permissible prescriptions electronically — eRx (40 percent requirement, does not apply to hospitals)
C 10	Use CPOE for medication orders directly entered by any licensed healthcare professional who can enter orders into the medical record per state, local, and professional guidelines. (30 percent for patients with at least one medication ordered through CPOE)
C 11	Implement drug-drug and drug-allergy interaction checks (functionality is enabled for these checks for the entire reporting period)
C 12	Implement capability to electronically exchange key clinical information among providers and patient authorized entities (Perform at least one test of EHR's capacity to exchange information)
C 13	Implement one clinical decision support rule relevant to specialty or high clinical priority along with and ability to track compliance for that rule.
C 14	Protect electronic health information created or maintained by the certified EHR technology through the implementation of appropriate technical capabilities (conduct or review a security risk analysis in accordance with the requirements and implement security updates as necessary)
C 15	Report ambulatory clinical quality measures to CMS or states (For 2011, provide aggregate numerator, denominator, and exclusions through attestation, 2012 submit electronically).

© Ingenix, Inc. 6

INGENIX.

Courtesy of Harris Care Tracker PM and EMR

Figure 5-1A   Stage 1 List of Core Requirements

The Menu Set Requirements – Final Regulation

ARRA EHR MEANINGFUL USE STAGE 1 REQUIREMENTS

CT #	MENU SET (must meet 5 of these)
M 16	Implement drug-formulary checks (generate at least one report for entire reporting period).
M 17	Incorporate clinical lab-test results into EHR as structured data (40 percent of all tests ordered with results in a positive/negative or numerical format).
M 18	Generate lists of patients by specific conditions to use for quality improvement, reduction of disparities, research, and outreach (generate at least one report with a list of patients with a specific condition)
M 19	Use certified EHR to identify patient-specific education resources and provide to patient if appropriate (10 percent requirement).
M 20	The eligible provider who receives a patient from another setting of care or provider of care or believes an encounter is relevant should perform medication reconciliation (50 percent requirement).
M 21	The eligible provider who transitions there patient to another setting of care or provider of care or refers their patient to another provider of care should provide summary care record for each transition of care and referral (50 percent requirement).
M 22	Capability to submit electronic data to immunization registries or Immunization Information Systems and actual submission in accordance with applicable law and practice (perform at least one test if the registry has the capability to receive electronically). NOTE: EP must complete one of Immunization or Syndromic Surveillance unless has an exception for both.
M 23	Capability to submit electronic syndromic surveillance data to public health agencies and actual transmission in accordance with applicable law and practice (perform at least one test unless public health agencies to not have the capacity to receive electronically) NOTE: Must complete one of Immunization or Syndromic Surveillance unless EP has an exception for both.
M24	Send appropriate reminders to patients per patient preference for preventative/follow up care during the 90 day reporting period for patients 65 and older or 5 years and younger (20 percent requirement).
M 25	Provide patients with timely electronic access to their health information, including laboratory results, problem list, medication list, and medication allergies within four business days of the information being available to the eligible provider (10 percent requirement).

INGENIX.

Courtesy of Harris Care Tracker PM and EMR

Figure 5-1B   Stage 1 Menu Set Requirements

Stage 2: Advance Clinical Processes

This stage focuses on expanding on Stage 1 criteria to encourage the use of health information technology (HIT) for continuous quality improvement at the point of care and the exchange of health information in the most structured format possible. Criteria for Stage 2 include:

- More rigorous health information exchange (HIE)
- Increased requirements for e-prescribing and incorporating lab results
- Electronic transmission of patient care summaries across multiple settings
- More patient-controlled data

Stage 3: Improved Outcomes

This stage focuses on the following:

- Promoting improvements in quality, safety, and efficiency
- Clinical decision support for national high-priority conditions
- Patient access to self-management tools
- Improving population health

Activity 5-1

Viewing the Meaningful Use Dashboard

The *Meaningful Use Dashboard* within Harris CareTracker PM tracks a provider's progress toward meeting the Medicare and Medicaid EHR Incentive Program reporting requirements for the core and menu set items. The dashboard displays a progress bar next to each of the measures that has a reporting requirement. **Figure 5-2A** illustrates a graphing screen of the core requirements for Dr. Olivia Sherman and

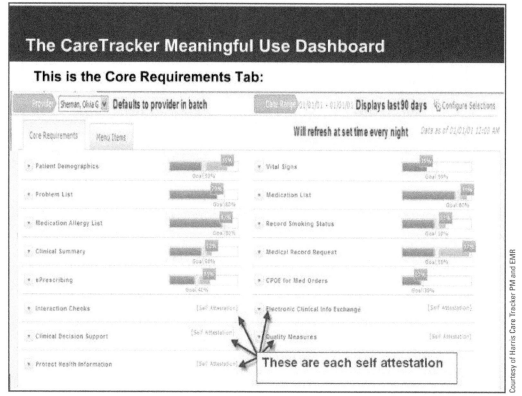

Figure 5-2A   Core Requirements for Dr. Olivia Sherman

Figure 5-2B illustrates the graphing features of the menu set requirements for Dr. Olivia Sherman. (Dr. Sherman is not a provider in our environment.)

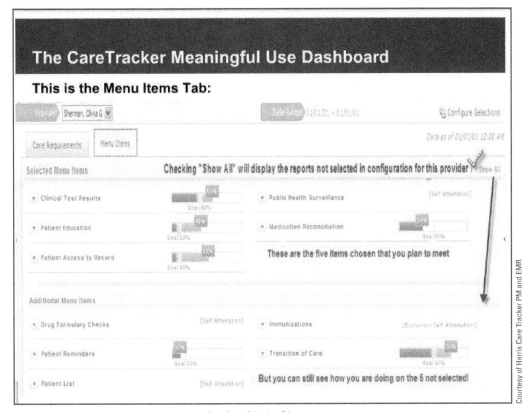

Figure 5-2B   Menu Requirements for Dr. Olivia Sherman

The dashboard's default date range is determined by when the provider begins the attestation period, or the date that begins the 90-day reporting period of meeting the core and menu measures listed previously. The dashboard calculates these measures over the previous 90 days. From the dashboard you can:

- Customize the requirements displayed on the dashboard for each participating provider
- View a status of a provider's progress for the last 90 days (percentages updated nightly)
- Hover over the percentage bar to review the data used to calculate the provider's percentage
- Click the *Menu Items* tab and then the drop-down arrow to download reference documents or run Key Performance Indicator (KPI) reports

Note: Any time you are working in the EMR side of Harris CareTracker, you need to make sure that "Compatibility View" settings is set to "Display intranet sites in Compatibility View." If you experience any functionality issues, please check your settings. (Refer to Best Practices for help.)

1. Click the *Home* module.

2. Click the *Meaningful Use* tab under the *Dashboard* tab (**Figure 5-3**). Harris CareTracker PM displays the *Meaningful Use Dashboard*.

3. From the *Provider* list, use the drop-down and select the name of the provider whose data you want to view. In this case, click on "Brockton, Anthony." Harris CareTracker PM displays the provider's percentages on the *Core Requirements* tab (**Figure 5-4**).

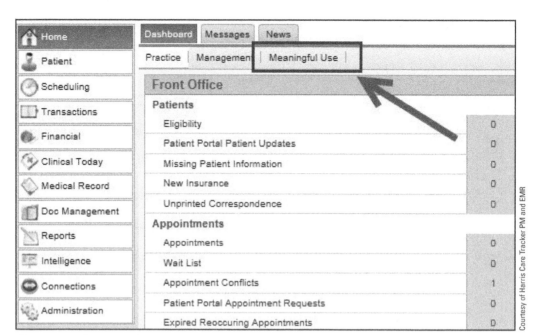

Figure 5-3   Meaningful Use Tab

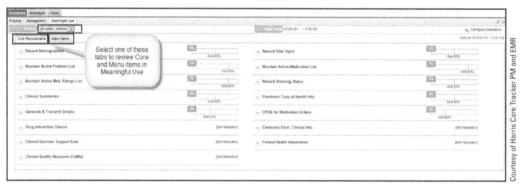

Figure 5-4   Dr. Brockton's Core Requirements

 Print a screenshot of the Core Requirements screen, label it "Activity 5-1A," and place it in your assignment folder.

4. Click the *Menu Items* tab to view the *Menu Items* requirements. On the *Menu Items* tab, select the *Show All* checkbox on the right-hand side of the screen to view any excluded requirements.

Print a screenshot of the Menu Items screen, label it "Activity 5-1B," and place it in your assignment folder.

PROFESSIONALISM CONNECTION

Providers will be impressed when you demonstrate knowledge of meaningful use and how and why the increased use of information technology will further improve patient safety, bring positive outcomes, and meet organizational goals.

FYI Because this is a training environment, you are only able to see the shell; no meaningful use statistics are available. **Figure 5-5** illustrates what a *Core Requirements* tab looks like in a fully functional environment.

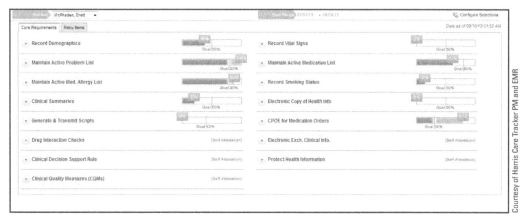

Figure 5-5   Core Requirements in a Fully Functional Environment

 ## Activity 5-2

Activating Care Management Items

The *Care Management* feature in Harris CareTracker PM and EMR allows practices to set clinical measures for health maintenance and disease management registries. The registries will assist with early identification of disease and early treatment. Keeping up-to-date with immunizations will help to prevent future disease and control costs associated with those diseases. This feature also assists in meeting some of the standards of meaningful use.

By default, clinical measures are turned off in Harris CareTracker PM and EMR. You need to activate the registries and measures you want to make available to the providers in your group. As you will observe, these registries will check to ascertain that the patient is up-to-date with preventive testing and immunizations. After activation, the registries and measures selected are included in the *Pt Care Management* application of the *Medical Record* module and the *Care Management* application of the *Clinical Today* module. Registries are repopulated with the *Clinical Today/Population Management* tab. Once activation occurs, anytime you open the patient's chart, you can see where he or she falls within the registries and help the patient to come into compliance with testing or procedures.

1. Click on the *Administration* module, and then click the *Clinical* tab.

2. Click the *Care Management Activation* link under the *Maintenances* heading (**Figure 5-6A**). Harris CareTracker PM and EMR launches the *Care Management Activation* application.

3. Select all of the measures and registries listed by selecting/clicking on all of the boxes. The checkboxes are dynamic and will auto-save on a single click. (A green "Saved" message appears briefly when each box is clicked to indicate the settings are saved [**Figure 5-6B**].)

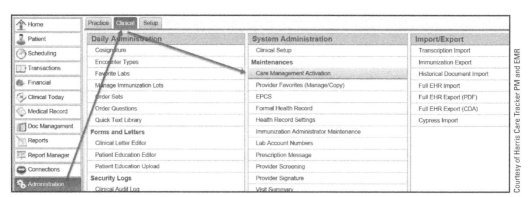

Figure 5-6A   Care Management Activation Link

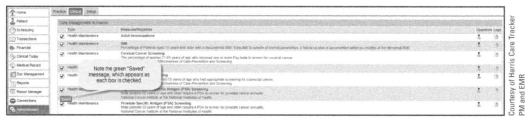

Figure 5-6B   Care Activation Measures and Registries

 Print the Care Management Activation screen, label it "Activity 5-2," and place it in your assignment folder.

4. Now click back on the *Clinical* tab and the *Care Management Activation* link to view the saved screen with all of the boxes checked.

PROFESSIONALISM CONNECTION

In case you did not make the connection, many of the disease prevention goals that you set for the patient are directly connected to meaningful use and the provider's core requirement percentages. When you are unable to get the patient to agree to these goals, it not only impacts the patient's health but the provider's meaningful use statistics. Because we are a "Pay for Performance" facility, it impacts the practice's bottom line as well.

PROFESSIONALISM CONNECTION

As you proceed with this chapter, you are going to learn a great deal about working in the patient's electronic medical record (EMR). You are very fortunate to enter the medical field at a time when technology is flourishing. Electronic medical records organize the patient's information so that you know exactly where each item is stored within the patient's chart. EMRs also help medical assistants stay on task and keep up with lab reports and prescription renewals. Your challenge is to embrace the training in this chapter so that you are able to fully navigate the patient's medical record in Harris CareTracker EMR. Consider how accurate documentation in a patient's EMR affects the billing and coding side of the practice and the revenue cycle.

OPERATOR PREFERENCES IN THE BATCH APPLICATION

Learning Objective 5: Set operator preferences in your Batch application.

Activity 5-3

Setting Operator Preferences in Your Batch Application

The *Batch* application in Harris CareTracker PM and EMR enables you to set up your operator preferences based on the workflow for your role. This reduces the number of clicks required to get from one application to the other, making navigation through Harris CareTracker easy. As a medical assistant working in a clinical capacity, you will want your screen to open in the *Clinical Today* module each time you log in to Harris CareTracker. Selecting the appropriate setting from the *Login Application* in your *Batch* preferences will take you directly to the *Clinical Today* module after logging in.

1. To set up operator preferences, with no patient in context, click *Batch* ▐ on the *Name Bar*. Harris CareTracker PM and EMR displays the *Operator Encounter Batch Control* dialog box.

2. Click on the *Edit* button.

3. Click on the drop-down arrow beside *Provider* and select "Dr. Raman," if he has not already been selected.

4. Click on the drop-down arrow beside *Resource* and select "Dr. Raman," if he has not already been selected.

5. Click on the drop-down arrow beside *Show Alerts* and select "Yes."

6. In the *Login Application* box, click on the drop-down arrow and select "Clinical."

7. Click on *Save*. Now every time you log into Harris CareTracker, you will be taken directly to the *Clinical Today* module.

8. Click "X" in the right-hand corner to close the dialog box.

NAVIGATING THE MEDICAL RECORD MODULE

Learning Objective 6: List major applications of the Clinical Today module.

Learning Objective 7: View daily appointments in Clinical Today.

Learning Objective 8: Perform check-in duties and track patients throughout their visits.

The *Medical Record* module is designed to mimic a paper chart and to follow the provider's normal workflow, facilitating effective EHR documentation for a patient. The module is accessed by pulling the patient into context on the *Name Bar* and then clicking the *Medical Record* module. If a patient has an appointment scheduled, you can click the patient name in the *Appointments* application (tab) of the *Clinical Today* module to launch the *Medical Record* module.

Patient Detail Bar

The *Patient Detail Bar* (**Figure 5-7**) displays the patient's picture (if available) and a summary of demographic, appointment, and clinical information. Additionally, your name displays as the operator who is currently accessing the patient's medical records. The Name Bar is located across the top of the CareTracker window and provides quick access to the most frequently used CareTracker applications.

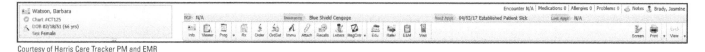

Courtesy of Harris Care Tracker PM and EMR

Figure 5-7   Patient Detail Bar

Patient Health History Pane

The *Patient Health History* pane (**Figure 5-8**) is a series of panes located to the left of the *Chart Summary* content in the *Medical Record* module that you can use to access different applications for reviewing, entering, and editing patient information such as diagnoses, medications, and more. The function of each pane is described in **Table 5-1**.

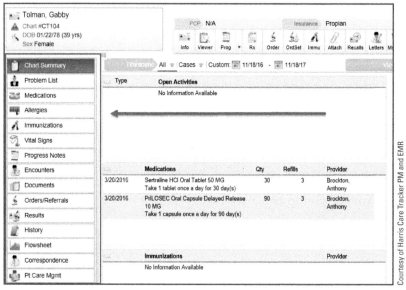

Figure 5-8   Patient Health History Pane

To familiarize yourself with these panes, go into Gabby Tolman's medical record, click out of the alert box, and click on each of the panes in the *Patient Health History* pane (e.g., click on *Chart Summary, Problem List, Medications*). You will learn the specifics of each pane to be used in future activities.

Table 5-1   Patient Health History Panes

PATIENT HEALTH HISTORY PANE	FUNCTION
Chart Summary	A view-only window displaying a summary of patient medical information.
Problem List	A list of chronic and ongoing patient problems.
Medications	Displays all prescribed medications for the patient.
Allergies	A list of patient allergies.
Immunizations	A list of immunizations given to the patient.
Vital Signs	Displays patient statistics such as height, weight, and blood pressure taken during each office visit or at home.
Progress Notes	Displays information about patient visits documented via quick text, point and click, dictation, or a combination of methods.
Encounters	Displays all patient encounters.
Documents	Displays all scanned or uploaded documents and voice recordings for the patient; for example, clinical documents, insurance cards, or identification cards.
Orders/Referrals	Displays test orders and referrals for the patient.
Results	Displays patient test results. Abnormal results display in red to help identify issues needing immediate attention.
History	Displays patient information such as the family, past medical and social history.
Flowsheet	Most commonly used for tracking vital statistics, diabetic insulin dosages, pain assessment, lab results, blood pressure, medication start and stop dates, physical assessment, and drug frequency.
Correspondence	Displays all *To Do*(s) for the patient and other communications such as patient education, recall, or collection letters provided or mailed to the patient.
Pt Care Mgmt	Displays a list of overdue preventive or maintenance items such as screening plans that need to be completed for the patient.

Clinical Toolbar

The *Clinical Toolbar* (**Figure 5-9**) is a convenient workflow tool that you can use to record information during a patient appointment. The toolbar can be found in *Medical Record* module and contains a series of tool buttons. The function of each button is described in **Table 5-2**.

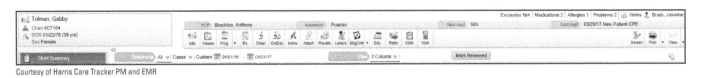

Courtesy of Harris Care Tracker PM and EMR

Figure 5-9   Clinical Toolbar

Table 5-2 Parts of the Clinical Toolbar

CLINICAL TOOL BUTTON	FUNCTION
Patient Information (Info)	The *Patient Information* window provides access to a patient's demographic, appointment, and other information.
Chart Viewer (Viewer)	The *Chart Viewer* provides a quick and easy way to access other applications when documenting a clinical encounter at the point of care.
Progress Note (Prog)	The *New Progress Notes* application helps you document the patient visits in various methods that include diagnosis-specific guidelines, provider-specific templates, pick list templates, dictation, or a combination of all.
Prescriptions (Rx)	The *Rx Writer* application (Surescripts® certified for prescription routing), uses the Surescripts® network to transmit electronic prescriptions directly to a selected pharmacy.
Order	The *Orders* application enables you to enter new orders and process orders by printing and sending to a clinical lab or by sending electronically via the Health Level 7 (HL7) interface.
Order Set (OrdSet)	The *Order Set* application enables you to group patient orders for a specific diagnosis or condition.
Immunizations (Immu)	The *Immunization* application facilitates documenting immunizations administered during a patient visit. Additionally, the application helps administer vaccinations from a "lot" and helps you manage information on immunization lots that pertain to the group.
Attachments (Attach)	The *Document Management Upload* application helps upload or scan documents that include anything from a letter to a medical report for the patient.
Recalls	The *Recall* application helps create patient reminders and letters for events such as annual physical exams, follow-up consultations, and lab tests.
Letters	The *Letters* application helps generate and print anything from a letter to a label for a patient by extracting information from the patient medical record.
Message Center (MsgCntr)	The *Messages* application facilitates patient-related communications with patients (if the patient is registered in Harris CareTracker's Patient Portal), office staff, and Harris CareTracker PM and EMR Support Department staff without having to pull or file a chart. There are three components in the Message Center: (1) New ToDo, (2) New Fax, and (3) New Mail.
Patient Education (Edu)	The *Patient Education* application gives you access to a comprehensive library of education material provided by Krames StayWell.
Referral (Refer)	The *Referral* application helps manage inbound and outbound referrals and authorizations.
E&M Evaluator (E&M)	The *E&M Evaluator* application helps identify the most appropriate E&M procedure (CPT®) code to use when charging for office visits and consultations.
Visits (Visit)	The *Visits* application helps capture information such as CPT® and ICD codes about the patient encounter.
Screen	The *Screen* feature enables you to check for drug interactions in real time for the patient in context.
Print	The *Print* feature helps export patient data into a PDF format in one- or two-column layout.
View	The *View* feature enables you to view the Clinical Log and the Continuity of Care Document (CCD) of the patient.

You will be using these tools throughout your training activities.

Activity 5-4
Viewing Appointments

At the start of each day, you will review the patient appointment list for the current workday. Some workers like to make copies of the schedule and have it close by for easy referencing; however, with Harris CareTracker PM and EMR, this information is just a screenshot away.

In Chapter 4, you scheduled three patients for future appointments. Now you will pull up some of these patients in *Clinical Today* and start working in the EMR portion of their records.

> **ALERT!** When you click on *Clinical Today*, the screen automatically defaults to the patients scheduled for the current date. For Activity 5-4, you will need the dates of the appointments you scheduled for patients in Chapter 4.

The *Appointments* application (**Figure 5-10**) consists of patient and non-patient appointments scheduled via the *Book* application in the *Scheduling* module.

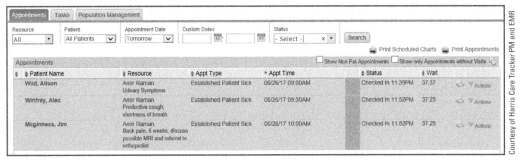

Figure 5-10 Appointment Screen in Clinical Today

To View Appointments:

1. Click on *Clinical Today*.

2. Click on the drop-down arrow under *Resource* and select "All."

3. Click on the drop-down arrow under *Patient* and select "All Patients."

4. Click on the drop-down arrow under *Appointment Date* and select "Custom."

5. Click on the calendar beside the first box under *Custom Dates* and select the date you scheduled your patient appointments in Chapter 4. (If you scheduled your patients on different dates, select the date that you scheduled Alison Wild.)

6. Click in the second box to the right of the calendar under *Custom Dates*. The date that you inserted in the first box should automatically populate in this box.

7. In the status box, click on the drop-down arrow and select "All" (**Figure 5-11**). **Note:** You may have to click back on the body of the *Status* box field for the drop-down to disappear.

8. Click on *Search*. (The *Appointments* screen with Ms. Wild's appointment should now appear along with any other appointments scheduled on this day.)

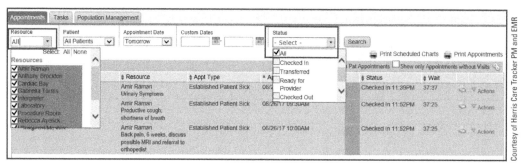

Figure 5-11   Select All

 Print a screenshot of your Appointments screen from Clinical Today. Label it "Activity 5-4" and place it in your assignment folder.

Activity 5-5

Transferring a Patient

In Chapter 4, you practiced checking in patients. Patients are typically checked in upon arrival. This cues the clinical staff that the patient is ready to be taken back to the exam room. This activity describes how to change a patient's status from "Checked In" to "Transferred." Transfer refers to the status of a patient when he or she has been taken to an exam room.

(A) Patient Alison Wild

1. Click on *Clinical Today*.

2. Match the search parameters to those set in Activity 5-4. Click *Search*.

3. Alison Wild's appointment should be listed in the *Appointments* window. Her current status is green, which means that she has already been checked in.

4. Change her status by clicking on the drop-down arrow to the left of the *Status* column and selecting "Transfer." (If the *Patient Alerts* popup box displays, close out of it by clicking on the "X" in the upper-right-hand corner.)

5. The *Patient Location* box will pop up. Select the radio button next to "Exam Room # 1."

6. Click *Select* (**Figure 5-12**). (**Note:** If there is nothing listed in the *Patient Location* box, review your Compatibility View setting (refer to Best Practices), and try again.)

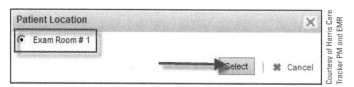

Figure 5-12   Patient Location Box

7. Ms. Wild's entry line should now be blue, indicating that she has been transferred to the exam room. The appropriate exam room number will now appear in the *Status* column (**Figure 5-13**).

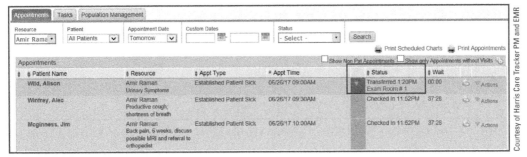

Figure 5-13   Exam Room Status Column

Repeat the steps in Activity 5-5 and transfer the following patients:

(B) Patient Alec Winfrey

(C) Patient Jim Mcginness

 Print a screenshot of the Exam Room Status Column. Label it "Activity 5-5" and place it in your assignment folder.

RETRIEVING AND UPDATING THE PATIENT'S ELECTRONIC MEDICAL RECORD

Learning Objective 9: Retrieve the patient's EMR and update sections within the patient health history panes.

Once the patient has been checked in and transferred to an exam room, you are ready to bring up his or her electronic medical record (EMR). In the case of Alison Wild, she is an established patient. Napa Valley Family Health Associates has transitioned from paper records to Harris CareTracker PM and Physician EMR. Because Ms. Wild has not been seen since the practice converted to electronic health records, her chart has not yet been converted. You will build her electronic chart from scratch in this chapter's activities.

PROFESSIONALISM CONNECTION

The status tab in the *Appointments* module within *Clinical Today* allows you to determine exactly where the patient is throughout the visit. It also tracks the length of time the patient spends in each area of the visit. If you happen to notice that the patient has been waiting particularly long in any area, even if it is not your assigned area, do a little investigating to establish the reason for the wait. Someone may have forgotten about the patient or may be tending to an emergency. Once you determine the reason for the wait, alert the patient and apologize for the delay. If the cirumstances causing the delay cannot be resolved within a reasonable period, offer the patient an opportunity to reschedule the appointment. The entire Napa Valley Family Health Associates staff is on the same team and need to support each other as well as the patient.

 ## Activity 5-6
Bringing Up the Patient's Chart

For activities related to this workbook, you will learn how to bring up the patient's chart and complete only certain functions required to continue with billing and coding activities. The clinical medical assistant will enter all of the patient's medical history, allergy information, medication list, vital signs, chief complaint, and preventive care and create flow sheets and growth charts. In addition, he or she will create the progress note (acting in a provider's role) and enter all necessary information. Entering clinical data will not be included in the activities of this workbook because we are focused only on the information that is needed to complete future billing and coding activities.

1. Click on *Clinical Today*.

2. In the *Appointments* screen within *Clinical Today*, bring up the date of Alison Wild's appointment. Be sure that *Resources* reflect "All." **Hint:** If you don't recall the date of the appointment, click on the *History* tab in the *Scheduling* module to locate the patient's appointment. Do not create a new encounter for this visit, only use the appointment/encounter previously scheduled.

3. Click on Ms. Wild's name. The patient's *Chart Summary* will open in a new window (**Figure 5-14**).

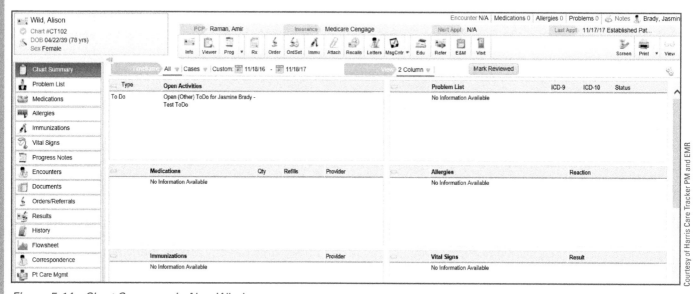

Figure 5-14   *Chart Summary in New Window*

 Print a screenshot of the Chart Summary in new window. Label it "Activity 5-6" and place it in your assignment folder.

Accessing the Patient Care Management Application

Learning Objective 10: Update the Patient Care Management application.

Activity 5-7

Accessing Patient Care Management Items

In Activity 5-2, you activated the *Care Management* feature in Harris CareTracker, which is <u>required</u> prior to using the *Patient Care Management* (*Pt Care Mgmt*) application. The *Patient Care Management* application is used to update information such as the due date or interval for a test/exam and to flag a test or exam that is refused by a patient as a proactive reminder tool to improve the care management process.

The patient is evaluated and moved to specific health maintenance and disease management registries based on measures that are activated within your group. The application helps manage the recurring preventive care items pertinent to a patient, flags overdue items, enables you to manually move the patient to a high-risk registry, and more. Additionally, you can view a list of care management items that are complete and pending for the patient by clicking the *Pt Care Mgt* link on the *Patient Health History* pane of the *Medical Record* module.

The care recommendations in the *Health Maintenance* and *Disease Management* registries are based on CDC and National Committee for Quality Assurance/Healthcare Effectiveness Data and Information Set (NCQA/HEDIS) guidelines.

Table 5-3 provides a description of each section within the *Patient Care Management* application.

Table 5-3 Sections within the Patient Care Management Application

SECTION	DESCRIPTION
Health Maintenance	This section displays all tests/exams that a patient is due for that are part of *Health Maintenance* registries.
Disease Management	This section displays all tests/exams that a patient is due for OR is required to have according to disease management measures. Click the *Expand* icon in the *Disease Management* section to view all items that are part of the disease management measure.

Courtesy of Harris CareTracker PM and EMR

Important: A patient is placed into a disease management measure only if the patient has an active diagnosis that triggers the ICD code rule.

To Access Patient Care Management Items:

1. If you are not in Alison Wild's medical record, access it by following the steps used in Activity 5-6.
   - Click on *Clinical Today*.
   - In the *Appointments* screen within *Clinical Today*, bring up the date of Alison Wild's appointment. Be sure that *Resources* reflect "All." **Hint:** If you don't recall the date of the appointment, click on the *History* tab in the *Scheduling* module to locate the patient's appointment. Do not create a new encounter for this activity; use only the appointment/encounter previously scheduled.
   - Click on Ms. Wild's name. The patient's *Chart Summary* will open in a new window (refer to Figure 5-14).

2. In the *Patient Health History* pane, click on the *Pt Care Mgmt* tab. Harris CareTracker EMR displays the *Patient Care Management* window with all health maintenance and disease management items completed for the patient (**Figure 5-15**). The list includes both pending and completed items. **Hint:** You must have completed Activity 5-2 for this feature to display.

3. Review the *Patient Care Management* window for Alison Wild.

 TIP You can remove a patient care management item from the list by clicking the *Deactivate* icon. The inactive item appears dimmed and you can select the *Show Inactive* checkbox to view the item.

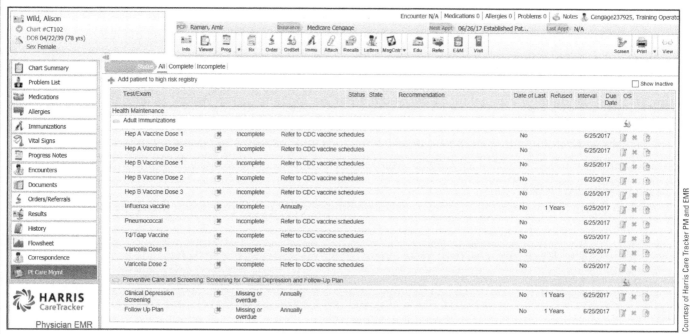

Figure 5-15 Patient Care Management Window

 Print a screenshot of the Patient Care Management list, label it "Activity 5-7," and place it in your assignment folder.

SPOTLIGHT Chapter 1 discussed that Napa Valley Family Health Associates is a "Pay for Performance" health care organization and that medical assistants in the practice are required to review patient Health and Disease Management registries prior to the patient's scheduled appointment. The clinical medical assistant will need to review this information and create a plan that identifies areas of concern and document steps he or she will take to bring the patient into compliance. The morning of the appointment, the plan should be shared with the provider. The provider will review the plan and make necessary adjustments. Electronic orders should be placed in the EMR prior to the appointment so that the "Catching Up" process can be performed throughout the visit. If the patient refuses any of the items listed in the plan, click on the *Edit* icon and signify that the patient refused the item. The reason for refusal should be entered in the *Notes* section of the dialog box. Sharing this information with the provider prior to patient examination gives the provider an opportunity to encourage those prevention or maintenance items that the patient refused. Consider how "Pay for Performance" relates to your position as a biller and coder.

CREATING PROGRESS NOTES

Learning Objective 11: Create and print a Progress Note.

 ## Activity 5-8

Accessing and Updating the Progress Notes Application

Progress notes are the heart of the patient record. They serve as a chronological listing of the patient's overall health status. Data pertaining to the findings from the visit are entered into the progress note. Most EMR software programs, including Harris CareTracker EMR, have progress note templates, copy and paste features, and automatic population tools, which make creating progress notes simplistic and efficient. The software also assists in promoting consistency from one provider to the next.

The *Progress Notes* application displays a list of notes recorded during each patient appointment and is required for medical, legal, and billing purposes. The note includes information such as the patient's history, medications, and allergies as well as a complete record of all that occurred during the visit. The application provides a quick and easy way to review and sign notes and helps identify notes that must be signed by a co-signer.

Note: Updating the *Progress Note* is typically a provider's responsibility and function; however, it is in the medical assistant's best interest to have knowledge and understanding of the *Progress Note*. Some practices use scribes. It is entirely possible that the medical assistant will then be responsible for recording the provider's findings. Although the entire activity is not required, the creation of the *Progress Note* (steps 1–6) is required and must be completed in order to complete later activities.

To Access and Update the Progress Notes Application:

(A) Patient Alison Wild

1. If you are not in Alison Wild's medical record, access it by following the steps used in Activity 5-6.

    - Click on *Clinical Today*.

    - In the *Appointments* screen within *Clinical Today*, bring up the date of Alison Wild's appointment. Be sure that *Resources* reflect "All." **Hint:** If you don't recall the date of the appointment, click on the *History* tab in the *Scheduling* module to locate the patient's appointment. Do not create a new encounter for this activity; use only the appointment/encounter previously scheduled.

    - Click on Ms. Wilds's name. The patient's *Chart Summary* will open in a new window (refer to Figure 5-14).

2. In the *Clinical Toolbar*, click the *Progress Notes* 📑 tab and select the encounter in context. If an encounter is in context, which in this case it is, Harris CareTracker EMR displays the *Progress Notes* template window (**Figure 5-16**). (**Note:** If documenting a progress note that is not based on an appointment, the *Encounter* dialog box displays, enabling you to create a new encounter. If you are getting an *Encounter* dialog box, it means that you did not have an encounter in context. Repeat step 1 if necessary.)

3. Alternatively, if the *Progress Notes* template window does not display, click on the date of the *Encounter* you want to make a progress note for. Then, beneath the *Progress Note* window, click *Edit*.

4. By default, the *View* field displays "Template." (Skip this box at this time.)

5. In the *Template* field, click on the drop-down arrow and select "IM OV Option 4 (v4) w/A&P" (see Figure 5-16). Complete the note by navigating through each tab as directed. (**Note:** You will be instructed to enter only minimal information to complete billing and coding activities.) The provider would ordinarily work in the progress note, but because the provider is not available you will be entering the information for the provider.

6. The *CC/HPI* tab will be showing on the right side of the screen. Place a check mark next to "Sick Visit" and "Established Patient" under *Chief Complaint*.

7. Review the note written regarding the patient's chief complaint. (**Note:** If the chief complaint was not yet entered, record "Urinary Symptoms" as the chief complaint in the *Other complaints* box.) The provider will expand a bit on the complaint by developing the History of Present Illness (HPI).

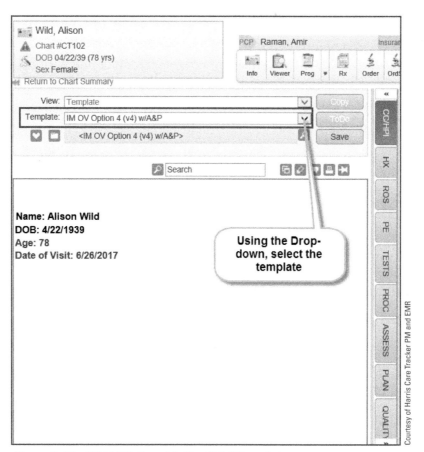

Figure 5-16   IM OV Option 4 (v4) w/A&P Template

8. While still in the *CC/HPI* tab, scroll down to the *HISTORY OF PRESENT ILLNESS* box and type the following:

"Patient has a history of UTI's (1–2 infections/year). Current episode includes frequency, urgency, and burning pain upon urination (6/10). Last UTI was approximately six months ago and resolved with a 10-day treatment of Bactrim DS." Your documentation should match **Figure 5-17**.

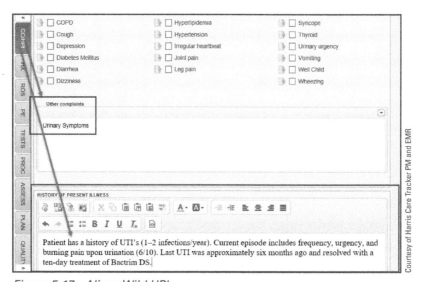

Figure 5-17   Alison Wild HPI

9. Click on *Save,* located in the template box in the middle of the screen (**Figure 5-18**).

10. Skip the *HX, ROS, PE, TESTS*, and *PROC* tabs.

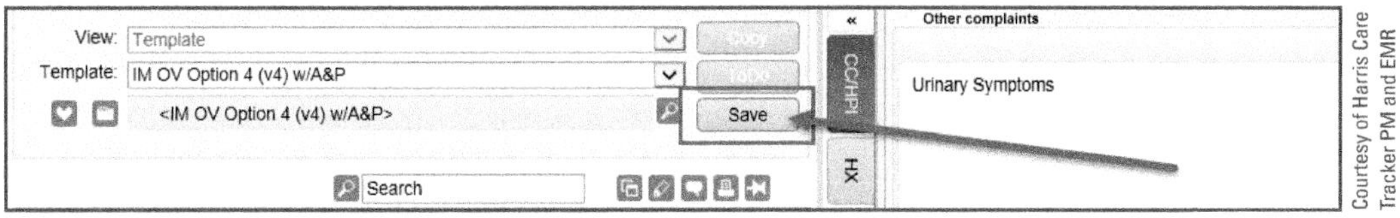

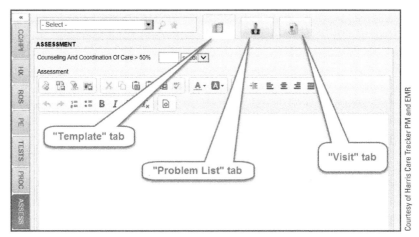

Figure 5-18   Save Button for Template Screen

11. Click on the *ASSESS* tab. By default, the *ASSESS* tab defaults to "Template." The other quick view tabs are the "Problem List" tab and the "Visit" tab (**Figure 5-19**).

Figure 5-19   Progress Note ASSESS Tab Icons

12. It was discovered during the exam that the patient has hypertension. The provider also diagnosed the patient with a urinary tract infection (UTI) and dysuria. You will be selecting only ICD-10 codes associated with the provider's diagnoses.

13. Click on the *Search* icon to the right of the *-Select-* drop-down menu at the top of the screen. In the *Diagnosis Search* window that pops up, enter "urinary tract infection" in the *Search Text* field and click the *Search* button. Click on "urinary tract infection" (ICD-10 code N39.0) in the results section of the *Diagnosis Search* window (note that it may have already been marked as a favorite diagnosis).

14. Search for and select "essential hypertension" (ICD-10 code I10).

15. Search for and select "recurrent and persistent hematuria" (ICD-10 code N02.9) and "dysuria" (ICD-10 code R30.0) as well. After selecting each diagnosis, scroll down to the bottom of the *ASSESS* tab, and see all selected codes listed under *Today's Selected Diagnosis*. Both the ICD-9 and ICD-10 versions of the code are listed (**Figure 5-20**).

16. Click *Save* to update the progress note with the *Assessment* information.

17. Click on the *PLAN* tab to record the provider's plans. Scroll down and document the following in the *Additional Plan Details* box (**Figure 5-21**):

a. Stat lab test—"Urinalysis dipstick panel by Automated test strip"

b. Send Urine out for lab test "Urinalysis microscopic panel [#volume] in urine by automated count"

c. Give patient educational handouts (1) Urinary Tract Infections in Women, and (2) What is Hematuria?

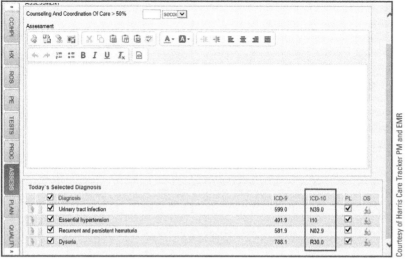

Figure 5-20   *Today's Selected Diagnosis*

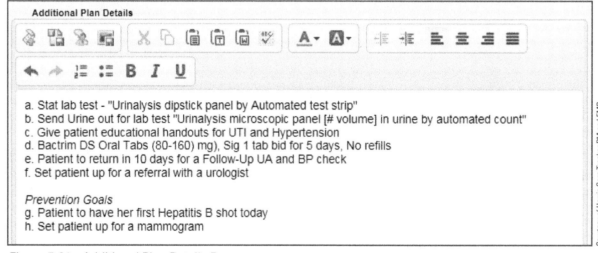

Figure 5-21   *Additional Plan Details Box*

d. Bactrim DS Oral Tabs (800–160 mg), Sig 1 tab bid for 5 days, No refills

e. Patient to return in 10 days for a Follow/Up UA and BP check

f. Set patient up for a referral with a urologist

PREVENTION GOALS:

g. Patient to have her first Hepatitis B shot today

h. Set patient up for a mammogram

PROFESSIONALISM CONNECTION

You will refer back to the *ASSESSMENT* and *PLAN* (A&P) noted in a patient's progress note when coding and billing. Keep this in mind as you move forward with billing-related tasks. You will need to be sure that all billable Evaluation and Management (E&M) and CPT® codes have been entered when saving the visit. Consider what would be the impact if all billable E&M and CPT® codes are not entered.

18. Click *Save*.

🖼 Click the orange Print 🖼 icon in the middle of the screen. The Clinical Note dialog box will open. Click the Print button to print a copy of the progress note. Label it "Activity 5-8A" and place it in your assignment folder.

19. Close out of the Printed Progress Note by clicking on the "X" in the upper-right-hand corner.

20. Click on the *Return to Chart Summary* link (in blue) at the top left of the screen to return to the patient's medical record.

Repeat Activity 5-8 for patients Alec Winfrey and Jim Mcginness. You will need to refer to the appointment dates for Alec Winfrey and Jim Mcginness that you scheduled in Chapter 4. You will also be referencing tables with information applicable to the patients' visits.

(B) Patient Alec Winfrey

Using the steps you learned in this chapter (Activities 5-6 and 5-8) and referencing information in **Table 5-4**, access Mr. Winfrey's medical record and create a progress note (update A&P). Mr. Winfrey is being seen today for a productive cough and shortness of breath.

Note: Select progress note template "IM OV Option 4 (v4) w/A&P."

Table 5-4 Alec Winfrey Medical Record and Progress Note

TAB	ENTRY
CC/HPI	*Chief Complaint*: Place a check mark in the "Sick Visit," "Established Patient," and "Cough" boxes. *Other complaints* box: Enter "Productive cough; shortness of breath" *History of Present Illness* box: Enter "Here today for cough that started 6 days ago and has gotten worse. Experiencing shortness of breath."
Skip the HX, ROS, PE, TESTS, and PROC Tabs	
ASSESS	*Diagnosis*: Pneumonia (J18.9) *Assessment* box: Enter "Bilateral Pneumonia."
PLAN	*Additional Plan Details* box: 1. CXR 2. CBC W Auto Differential panel in Blood 3. EKG 4. Ibuprofen 800 mg oral now and instruct for every six hours while awake 5. Return visit in two days 6. Seek treatment in the ED or UC if symptoms worsen 7. Zithromax Z-Pack, one as directed

🖼 After entering all of the information provided in Table 5-4, print a progress note, label it "Activity 5-8B," and place it in your assignment folder.

(C) Jim Mcginness

Using the steps you learned in this chapter (Activities 5-6 and 5-8) and referencing information in
Table 5-5, access Mr. Mcginness's medical record and create a progress note (update A&P). Mr. Mcginness
is being seen today for a productive cough and shortness of breath.

    Note: Select progress note template "IM OV Option 4 (v4) w/A&P."

Table 5-5   Jim Mcginness Medical Record and Progress Note

TAB	ENTRY
CC/HPI	*Chief Complaint:* Place check marks in the "Sick Visit," "Established Patient," and "Back Pain" boxes. *Other complaints* box: Enter "Back pain, 3 weeks, discuss possible MRI and referral to Orthopedist. Patient continues to have intense lower back pain following an injury three weeks ago while lifting heavy boxes at home." *History of Present Illness* box: Enter "Patient picked up a large box at home approximately three weeks ago and immediately felt a sharp pain in his lower back. Pain started at a 5/10 and subsided to a 2/10 the following day. Pain has been steadily increasing and is now an 8/10. Patient describes pain as tight and continuous. Activity makes pain worse; sitting still in an upright position makes it feel slightly better. Patient has been taking Tylenol and using a heating pad since onset (little relief). Patient denies any numbness, tingling, or pain that radiates down either leg or previous low back pain or trauma."
Skip the Hx, ROS, PE, TESTS, and PROC Tabs	
ASSESS	*Diagnosis:* Low back pain M54.5 *Assessment:* Somatic Dysfunction-Lumbar, Pelvis
PLAN	*Additional Plan Details* box: 1. Refer for LS MRI 2. Referral to Orthopedist 3. Oxycodone-Acetaminophen 10–325 mg tabs 4. Follow-up appointment when MRI is complete

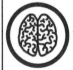 **After entering all of the information provided in Table 5-3, print a progress note, label it "Activity 5-8C,"
and place it in your assignment folder.**

CRITICAL THINKING   At the beginning of this chapter, you were asked to keep in mind how your position as a medical assistant may be impacted by meaningful use, and how you will be able to assist both providers and patients in meeting these goals. Having completed your studies and activities, describe how you see your role in the practice as an advocate for both the provider and patients. How will you incorporate meaningful use and patient care management in your daily activities? How are your duties as a billing/coding professional impacted by meaningful use?

CRITICAL THINKING You were also challenged to embrace the EMR training in this chapter so that you are able to fully navigate the patient's medical record in Harris CareTracker EMR. Now that you have completed many detailed clinical tasks, did you find the transition from administrative to clinical duties to be seamless? Were there any particular activities that were challenging? What steps did you take to work through the tasks? Does the amount of information needed to accurately record patient information and patient care help with your understanding of the roles of health care providers and the health care system overall? What impacts do clinical tasks have on billing/coding responsibilities? Explain your thoughts and conclusions.

 CASE STUDY
Case Study 5-1

Repeat Activity 5-7 and Access the Patient Care Management application for patient Harriet Oshea.

🖳 **Print a screenshot of the Patient Care Management list, label it "Case Study 5-1," and place it in your assignment folder.**

Completing
the Visit

6

Learning Objectives

1. View and resolve open encounters and unsigned notes by completing and capturing the visit.
2. Access, view, sign, and print a progress note.

Real-World Connection

In this chapter, you will learn to complete the visit and how documentation in both PM and EMR will affect your responsibilities as a biller and coder. You will also learn to capture a visit (selecting procedure and diagnosis codes for the patient's visit). The electronic health record makes orders and visit capture a seamless process. You will refer to the A&P of the progress note to review whether all billable services have been captured.

Consider this scenario: The provider (or MA depending on workflows) selected a service code (Z00.00) that is not covered by the patient's insurance (Medicare). How would you resolve this issue?

a. Confront the provider/MA who entered the code and ask why he or she used that code.
b. Confront the provider/MA and tell him or her that Z00.00 is never covered by Medicare and that this is the second time this week a claim was rejected for the same code.
c. Confront the provider/MA and tell him or her that you have seen the same rejection more than once on Medicare patients. Ask the provider/MA for input as to why that might be.
d. Offer an explanation of codes that are often rejected and schedule an in-service training for all providers/ staff.
e. Go to the billing supervisor first to let him or her know of the claim rejection and have him or her handle it.
f. Handle the code change yourself and do not notify the clinical MA or provider.

Discuss this scenario with your class. How billers and coders choose to handle these types of situations reflects on their knowledge and professionalism.

Before you begin the activities in this chapter, refresh your memory on working with Harris CareTracker by referring back to the Best Practices list on page xiv of this workbook. Following best practices will help you complete work quickly and accurately.

COMPLETING A VISIT FOR BILLING

Learning Objective 1: View and resolve open encounters and unsigned notes by completing and capturing the visit.

Learning Objective 2: Access, view, sign, and print a progress note.

Activity 6-1

Access the Progress Notes Application

Progress notes are the heart of the patient record. They serve as a chronological listing of the patient's overall health status. Data pertaining to the findings from the visit are entered into the progress note. Most EMR software programs, including Harris CareTracker EMR, have progress note templates, copy and paste features, and automatic population tools, which make creating progress notes simplistic and efficient. The software also assists in promoting consistency from one provider to the next.

The *Progress Notes* application displays a list of notes recorded during each patient appointment and is required for medical, legal, and billing purposes. The note includes information such as the patient's history, medications, and allergies as well as a complete record of all that occurred during the visit. To navigate and view the progress notes listed in a patient's medical record:

- Click the *Next* and *Previous* buttons on the bottom of the *Progress Note* window to navigate through the list of notes (**Figure 6-1**).

- Click the *Expand/Collapse* ✚ icon in the upper-right-hand corner of your screen to maximize the view for readability.

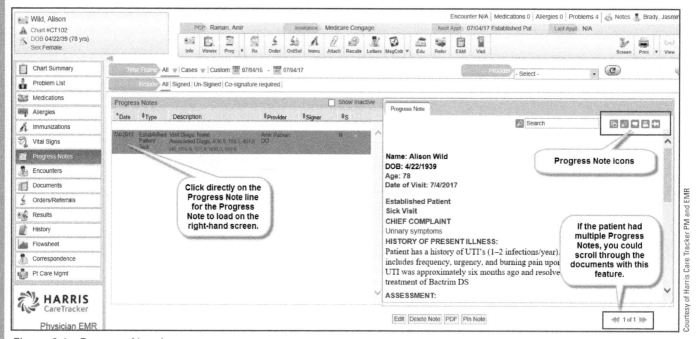

Figure 6-1   *Progress Note Icons*

Note: Updating the *Progress Note* is typically a provider's responsibility and function; however, it is in the medical assistant's best interest to have knowledge and understanding of the *Progress Note*.

 TIP   Important!! Complete and sign all progress notes before any billing information is submitted to the payers.

To Access the Progress Notes Application:

1. There are several ways to access the *Medical Record* module. Use one of the following methods:

    a. Pull the patient Alison Wild into context, and click the *Medical Record* module.

    b. Click on *Clinical Today*.

    • In the *Appointments* screen within *Clinical Today*, bring up the date of Alison Wild's appointment. Be sure that *Resources* reflect "All." **Hint:** If you don't recall the date of the appointment, click on the *History* tab in the *Scheduling* module to locate the patient's appointment. Do not create a new encounter for this activity, use only the appointment/encounter previously scheduled.

2. Select the date of the patient's appointment that you scheduled in Chapter 4.

3. In the *Patient Health History* pane in the medical record, click *Progress Notes*.

4. The *Progress Notes* window displays with a list of signed and unsigned notes for the patient (**Figure 6-2**).

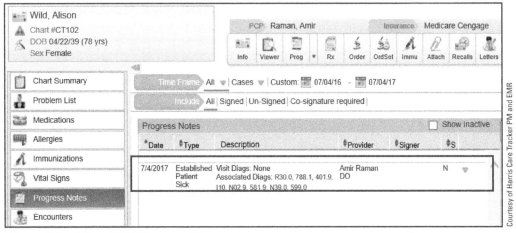

Figure 6-2   Alison Wild Progress Note

5. (FYI) The workflow would be that all tasks assigned by the provider for Alison Wild's encounter created in Chapter 5 have been completed. To confirm, click on the progress note on the left-hand side of the screen, and then click *Edit* at the bottom right side of the screen. This will launch the progress note. Select the *PLAN* tab to confirm that all orders, immunizations, referrals, and educational materials ordered in the A&P have been completed (**Figure 6-3**).

6. You note that the patient is to return in 10 days for a follow-up UA and blood pressure check. Make a follow-up appointment for Alison Wild with Dr. Raman for 10 days from her original encounter (**Figure 6-4**). (Refer to Chapter 4, Activity 4-1, if you need to review the instructions for scheduling an appointment.)

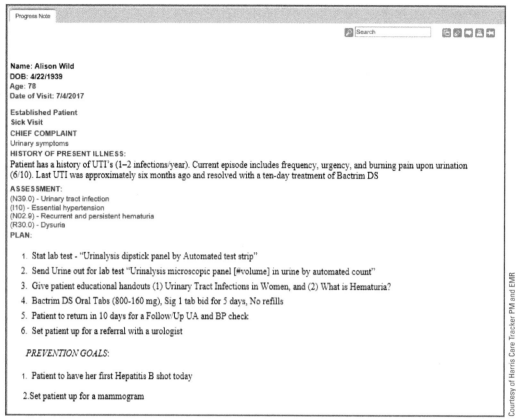

Figure 6-3   Additional Plan Details for Alison Wild

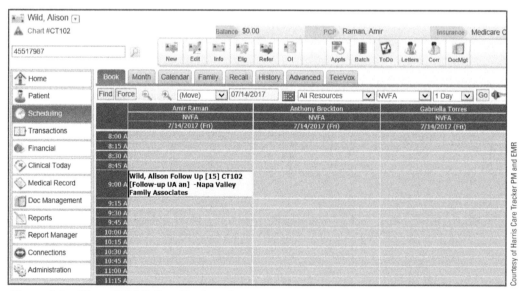

Figure 6-4   Alison Wild Follow-Up Appointment

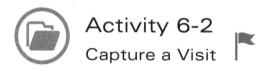

Activity 6-2
Capture a Visit

In Chapter 5, you completed much of the patient work-up to the point of completing and printing the progress note. In order for a patient visit to be billable, any open encounters must be resolved and the visit must be completed and the note signed. The provider is the person who is responsible for signing the progress note; however, to enhance your understanding of workflows in the EMR, you will be completing the visit, resolving open encounters, and electronically signing the note.

To generate claims, charges must be captured for the patient's appointment. The *Visit* application allows you to capture charges and enter procedure, NDC, and diagnosis codes for a patient's appointment. Visits can be entered into Harris CareTracker PM and EMR by one of the following methods:

- Left-click on a patient's appointment in the *Book* application and select *Visit* from the pop-up mini-menu.

- Pull a patient into context, click the *Appts* button in the *Name Bar,* pull the appointment into context, and select *Visit* from the *Actions* menu.

- Click the *Appointments* link under the *Appointments* section of the *Dashboard* tab in the *Home* module, pull the patient appointment into context, and then select *Visit* from the *Actions* menu.

- Click the *Visits* link from the *Actions* drop-down list for a patient listed in the *Appointments* application of the *Clinical Today* module.

- Click the *Visit* icon on the *Clinical Toolbar* within the *Medical Record* module.

The *Visit* window contains a number of applications, but to save a visit you only need to enter the procedure and diagnosis code(s). Please note that a visit can only be edited prior to becoming a charge. For our first *Visit* activity, refer to patient Alec Winfrey's appointment that you scheduled in Chapter 4 with Dr. Raman. Access the *ASSESS* and *PLAN* tabs in the *Progress Note* (**Figure 6-5**) and capture the *Visit.* Mr. Winfrey is being seen today for a productive cough and shortness of breath.

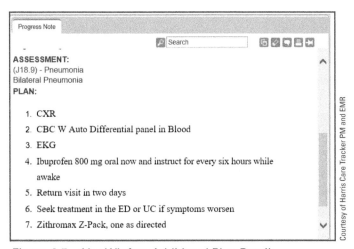

Figure 6-5   Alec Winfrey Additional Plan Details

To Capture a Visit:

6-2(A): Patient Alec Winfrey

1. Click the *Scheduling* module. Harris CareTracker PM and EMR opens the *Book* application by default.

2. Move the schedule to display the date of service for which you want to confirm an appointment. This can be done by manually entering the date in the *Date* box, by clicking the *Calendar* icon, or by selecting a time period from the *Move* list. (Use the date from Activity 4-1 in the date box.)

3. You will need to set the *Resources* field (just to the right of the calendar) to "All Resources" using the drop-down to select "All Resources" in order for the full schedule and all providers to display.

4. Click *Go*.

5. Left-click the appointment for which you want to enter visit information and select *Visit* from the mini-menu (select Alec Winfrey's appointment). The application displays the *Visit* window (**Figure 6-6**). When you first bring up the *Visit* window, it automatically displays the procedures section (*Procedures* tab located at the top left of the window).

Procedures	Diagnosis	Visit Summary						EncoderPro.com

Pt Name Winfrey, Alec (M)		**PCP** Raman, Amir		**Admit Date** N/A		**Notes**
DOB 7/8/1965 (51 yrs)		**Ref Provider** Shinaman, Richard		**Last Surgery Date** N/A		
Primary Ins Century		**Case Ins** Century		**Next Appointment** None		**Complaint** Productive coug…

Procedure Search: [   ] 🔍

☑ 85025 - Complete Cbc W/Auto Diff Wbc [1]   ☑ 36415 - Routine Venipuncture [1]

OFFICE VISIT EST PTS	Mod	Units	OFFICE PROCEDURES	Mod	Units	PREVENTIVE MEDICINE EST	Mod	Units
☐ 99212 Office Outpatient Visit 10 Min	[ ]	[1]	☐ 93000 Ecg Routine Ecg W/Least 12 Lds	[ ]	[1]	☐ 99395 Periodic Preventive Med Est Pa	[ ]	[1]
☑ 99213 Office Outpatient Visit 15 Min	[ ]	[1]	☐ G0102 Pros Cancer Screening; Digtl R	[ ]	[1]	☐ 99396 Periodic Preventive Med Est Pa	[ ]	[1]
☐ 99214 Office Outpatient Visit 25 Min	[ ]	[1]	☐ 94760 Noninvasive Ear/Pulse Oximetry	[ ]	[1]	☐ 99397 Periodic Preventive Med Est Pa	[ ]	[1]
☐ 99215 Office Outpatient Visit 40 Min	[ ]	[1]	☐ J7650 Isoetharine Hci Inhal Thru Dme	[ ]	[0]	PREVENTIVE MEDICINE NEW	Mod	Units
OFFICE VISIT NEW PTS	Mod	Units	☐ 94620 Pulmonary Stress Testing Simpl	[ ]	[1]	☐ 99384 Initial Preventive Medicine Ne	[ ]	[1]
☐ 99201 Office Outpatient New 10 Minut	[ ]	[1]	☐ D7911 Complicated Suture-Up To 5 Cm	[ ]	[1]	☐ 99385 Initial Preventive Medicine Ne	[ ]	[1]
☐ 99202 Office Outpatient New 20 Minut	[ ]	[1]	☐ 93225 Xtrnl Ecg < 48 Hr Recording	[ ]	[1]	☐ 99386 Initial Preventive Medicine Ne	[ ]	[1]
☐ 99203 Office Outpatient New 30 Minut	[ ]	[1]	☐ V5008 Hearing Screening	[ ]	[1]	☐ 99387 Initial Preventive Medicine Ne	[ ]	[1]
☐ 99204 Office Outpatient New 45 Minut	[ ]	[1]	☐ 3210F Group A Strep Test Performed	[ ]	[1]	INJECTIONS	Mod	Units
RADIOLOGY	Mod	Units	OTHER SERVICES	Mod	Units	☐ 90471 Imadm Prq Id Subq/Im Njxs 1 Va	[ ]	[1]
☑ 71020 Radiologic Exam Chest 2 Views	[ ]	[1]	☐ Q0091 Screen Pap Smear; Obtain Prep	[ ]	[1]	☐ 90658 Influenza Virus Vaccine Split	[ ]	[1]
☐ 72100 Radex Spine Lumbosacral 2/3 Vi	[ ]	[1]	☐ 88143 Cytp C/V Flu Auto Thin Mnl Scr	[ ]	[1]	☐ G0008 Administration Of Influenza Vi	[ ]	[1]

Figure 6-6   Alec Winfrey Visit Window (Procedures Tab)

6. The *Procedures* screen contains a list of procedure codes that mirror the CPT® codes on the encounter form. Place and verify that the checkboxes next to each code associated with the patient's appointment are selected. Select CPT® codes 99213, 71020, 36415, and 85025 for this visit. (**Note:** If no *Visit* had yet been entered for the patient, the encounter form would display with no checkboxes next to procedure or diagnose codes. If you see the code you want to select for the *Visit*, you can select the checkbox next to the code. Alternatively, you could enter either a code or key term in the *Procedure Search* box and click *Search* to locate the desired code.)

Source: Current Procedural Terminology © 2017 American Medical Association.

TIP If you need to search for a CPT® code:

- Enter a partial code, complete code, or a keyword in the *Procedure Search* field, and then click the *Search* icon. The application opens the *Procedure Search* window.
- *(Optional)* To search for an NDC Code, select *NDC Code* from the *Search Type* list and then click *Search*.
- Click on the desired procedure to select it. The codes selected from the search are added to the patient's *Visit* window and there is no limit to the number of codes you can select.

- **Note:** If a code is not listed on the NVFHA encounter form, you will receive a pop-up warning that the code was not found. This does not mean it is an invalid code, only that it is not one of the codes included on the existing encounter form. You will still be able to add the code manually, although you may be prompted to enter the associated fee as well. If no fee is associated with the charge, you will make a note in the *Visit Summary/Billing Notes* section.

PROFESSIONALISM CONNECTION

As biller and coder, you must select and enter all service/procedure and diagnosis codes. If the codes are not already pre-populated in the A&P, do you know where to find them? **Hint:** For each of the codes you were instructed to select, there is a narrative in the A&P. For example:

- 99213 = Established patient, sick visit (15 minutes)
- 71020 = Bilateral Chest X-Ray
- 36415 = Venipuncture
- 85025 = Laboratory: CBC W Auto Differential panel in Blood

If you had not checked the verbiage in the patient's A&P of the progress note, you may have missed all the codes related to services. Consider this as you move through activities related to billing and coding.

7. Enter any modifiers in the *Mod* field next to each selected procedure code, if applicable. (No modifier is required.)

8. If needed, enter the number of units in the *Units* field for each selected procedure code. (Number of units is "1" per CPT® code for this activity [as noted in Figure 6-6].)

9. Click the *Diagnosis* tab in the *Visit* window. The application displays the *Diagnosis* application.

10. The *Diagnosis* screen displays a list of codes that mirror the ICD codes on the encounter form. Select the checkbox next to each code associated with the patient's appointment. Because the type of pneumonia (organism) is not known at this stage, you will select ICD-10 code J18.9. The checkbox next to the diagnosis code will now be selected as in **Figure 6-7**. (**Note:** You can also scroll down the *Diagnosis* screen, locate the ICD-10 code, and place a check mark next to the selected diagnosis.)

TIP If you need to search for a diagnosis code:

- Enter a partial code, a complete code, or a keyword in the *Diagnosis Search* field, and then click the *Search* icon. The application opens the *Diagnosis Search* window.
- Click on the desired ICD-10 code to select it. The codes selected from the search are added to the patient's *Visit* window.

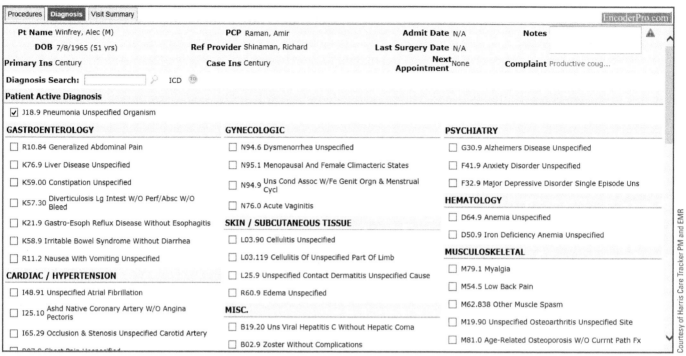

Figure 6-7   Alec Winfrey Diagnosis Codes

11. Click the *Visit Summary* tab in the top left corner of the *Visit* window. Harris CareTracker PM displays a summary of the visit information.

12. To check out the patient directly from the *Visit* application, select the *Check out Patient?* checkbox (**Figure 6-8**) at the bottom of the screen.

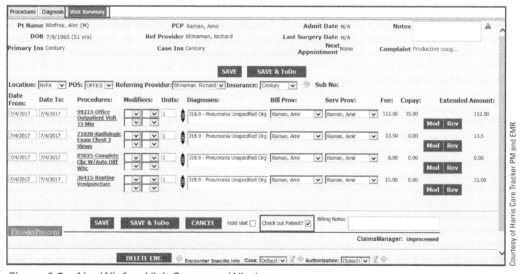

Figure 6-8   Alec Winfrey Visit Summary Window

13. Review the screen (see Figure 6-8) and verify the accuracy of the information including the *Location*, *Place of Service (POS)*, *Referring Provider*, *Insurance*, *Billing*, and *Servicing Provider*.

14. (If applicable) To link the visit to a case, you would select a case from the *Case* list. (No *Case* number is associated with this visit.)

15. Select an authorization number from the *Authorization* list, if applicable (not applicable in this activity).

16. In the *Billing Notes* section, leave blank.

17. From the *Billing Type* list, select the billing type "Professional" at the bottom of the *Visit* screen (**Figure 6-9**).

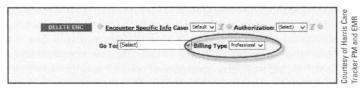

Figure 6-9   Billing Type-Professional

18. *(Optional)* Click *EncoderPro.com* to obtain coding information from *EncoderPro*. This information can be used as a guide to correct the visit information.

🖫 **Print the Visit Summary screen. Label it "Activity 6-2A," and place it in your assignment folder.**

19. Click *Save* at the top or bottom of the screen. Once you hit *Save*, you will receive a pop-up message (**Figure 6-10**) stating "An error occurred connecting to Claims manager. Transaction saved." You must *wait* for this error message before continuing with the activity. Once you receive the error message, click *OK* on the pop-up.

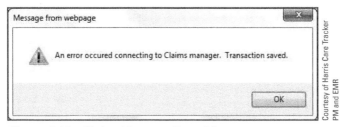

Figure 6-10   ClaimsManager Error Message

20. When the visit is saved, the coding information is sent to *ClaimsManager* for screening. In addition, Harris CareTracker PM and EMR automatically checks out the patient on the schedule and a check mark appears next to the patient's name confirming that the visit has been captured. Your *Claims-Manager* feature is not active in your student version of Harris CareTracker which is why you receive the error message, but the visit is saved for this activity and future billing activities.

6-2 (B): Patient Jim Mcginness:

Repeat Activity 6-2 (Capture a Visit) using the information that follows. Refer to the encounter you created for Mr. Mcginness in Chapter 5. Mr. Mcginness is being seen today for back pain.

    a.   *CPT® Code*: 99213

        Source: Current Procedural Terminology © 2016 American Medical Association.

    b.   *ICD-10 Codes*: M54.5; M99.03; M99.05

🖫 **After saving the visit charges, print a screenshot of the completed visit summary and label it "Activity 6-2B."**

PROFESSIONALISM CONNECTION

Using Real Time Adjudication (RTA) is becoming more commonplace as medical practices strive to remain financially viable. This is especially true for specialty practices that provide services in addition to office visits (e.g., orthopedic outpatient procedures). RTA is a relatively new concept and practices and staff may struggle to incorporate it into their billing practices. RTA does not make much, if any, change to the way an HMO insurance is handled. HMOs typically have a copay amount for office visits, hospital visits, and so on that does not vary, and patients have always paid their copay upon check-in.

RTA especially affects the workflow and common practice for Medicare and PPO insurance. Medicare and most PPOs typically have an 80/20 split. This means that once the claim is submitted, it is adjusted by Medicare or the PPO insurance company to the contracted rate for the service(s) billed. After applying the contracted rate, the insurance pays 80% (after any initial annual deductible or out-of-pocket patient requirements, if any, have been satisfied), and then the patient is responsible for the remaining 20%. Although some PPOs also have a copay requirement or a different insurance/patient split (e.g., $20 copay and 70/30 split), patients with Medicare and PPO insurance have been accustomed to waiting for the EOB from their insurance company to advise them of the contracted amount, what was paid by insurance, and what balance (e.g., 20%) the patient owes. The patient then receives a bill from the provider/practice. As practices incorporate RTA into their workflows, they will need to be sensitive to patient concerns when asking for patients to pay their "share" at the time of the visit.

Applying RTA practices to larger amounts, such as specialty outpatient services, may be even more challenging. Imagine a patient who needed an emergency outpatient orthopedic procedure and instead of getting a call from the provider's office the next day to see how he or she was doing, the call instead was to advise the patient how much his or her share of the bill was going to be. Consider how you, as a biller and coder, would incorporate this new policy of advising patients of any estimated balance due to the practice. Discuss with the class the concept of using RTA and various dialogs to use with patients.

Activity 6-3
Resolve an Open Encounter

In Harris CareTracker PM and EMR, you have the option to save a visit directly as a charge. This eliminates the additional steps of either navigating to the *Charge* screen to save the charge from the previously created visit or from having to save *Bulk Charges* via the *Missing Encounters* link on the *Dashboard*.

An encounter is an interaction with a patient on a specific date and time. Encounter types include visits, phone calls, referrals, results of a test, and more. The *Open Encounters* application displays a list of appointment-based "visit" type of encounters that do not have a corresponding clinical note and also identifies patients who have a clinical note for a specific date of service but no encounter billed for that same date. Additionally, the *Open Encounters* application displays customized encounters that require billing or a signed note. The *Open Encounters* application is accessible from the following locations:

- *Home* module > *Dashboard* tab > *Open Encounters* link (*Clinical* section) (**Figure 6-11**)

- *Clinical Today* module > *Tasks* tab > *Open Encounters* (from the *Tasks* menu on the right side of the window) (**Figure 6-12**)

Courtesy of Harris Care Tracker PM and EMR

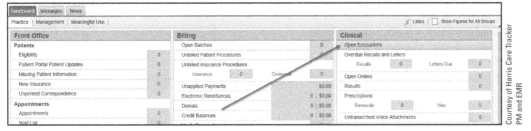

Figure 6-11 Open Encounters Link on Dashboard Tab

Courtesy of Harris Care Tracker PM and EMR

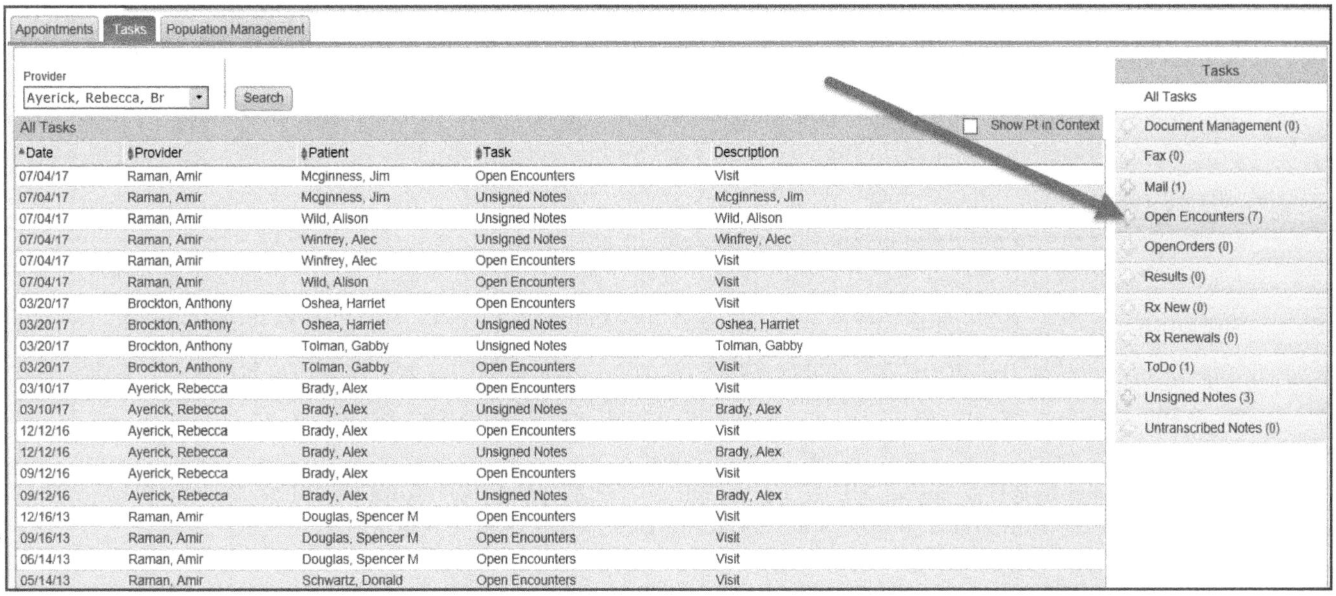

Figure 6-12 Open Encounters from the Clinical Today Module

- An alternative method is to click the *Clinical Today* module and *Tasks* tab and view open encounter tasks in the *All Tasks* window. You can sort on the *Tasks* column to easily identify open encounter tasks.

The *Open Encounters* application helps resolve appointment-based "visit" type of encounters by entering the visit information, reviewing, transcribing (if the note contains an untranscribed file), signing the note, and then billing. Patient Alison Wild is being seen today for urinary symptoms.

To Resolve an Open Encounter:

1. Access the *Open Encounters* application from the *Home* module > *Dashboard* tab > *Open Encounters* link (*Clinical* section). If the encounter you are looking for does not display, use the drop-down feature next to *Provider*, select *All*, and then click the *Change Resource* (search) (C).

2. Find the encounter you want to resolve (**Figure 6-13**). (Locate the encounter you created for Alison Wild.)

Courtesy of Harris Care Tracker PM and EMR

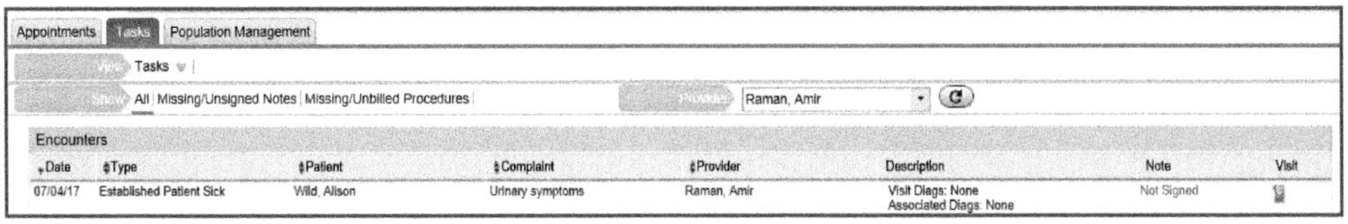

Figure 6-13 Alison Wild Open Encounter

3. Under the *Note* column, click the *Not Signed* link. The *Progress Note* application displays, enabling you to complete and sign the note if instructed.

4. As best practice, you would confirm (resolve) that all items in the *A&P* for the encounter have been completed. This is the opportunity for the medical assistant to complete any orders, education materials, future appointments, etc.

5. Do *not* sign the note at this time.

6. (FYI) As best practice, you would perform an eligibility check on the patient before saving the visit.

7. Click on the *Visit* 🔲 icon in the *Clinical Toolbar*. The *Visit* application will display. **Note**: You may have to click back on the *Home* module for the *Visit* tab to display.

8. You would normally enter the codes as noted by the provider (Z00.00 and 90746) (**Figure 6-14**), but you determine upon reviewing the patient's A&P and results of eligibility check that you need to do further research. You determine that Z00.00 is an incorrect code for Medicare patients and should be coded 99213 for an established patient, sick visit. In addition, you noted on the A&P that the patient had a urinalysis; therefore, you would need to add a CPT® code for specimen handling (99000). Although the Hep B vaccine CPT® code was entered (90746), there is also a CPT® code for a fee for the injection (90471). Therefore, you will resolve the open encounter by selecting the following codes:

    • In the *Procedures* tab, select CPT® codes 99213; 90746; 99000; and 90471.

      Source: Current Procedural Terminology © 2016 American Medical Association.

    • In the *Diagnosis* tab, select ICD-10 codes N39.0, R30.0, and I10. (**Note**: Scroll down the *Diagnosis* screen and confirm that all the selected diagnoses have been checked.)

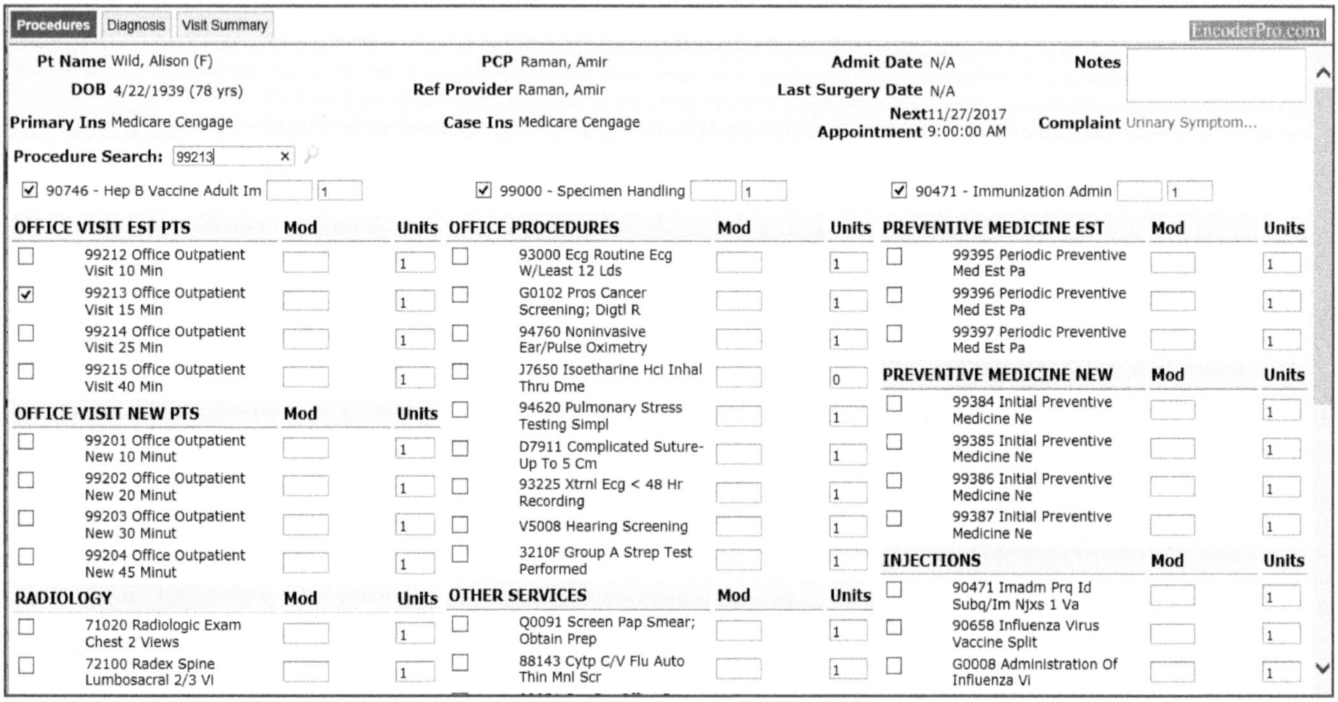

Figure 6-14 *Alison Wild Procedures Screen*

9. Click on the *Visit Summary* tab. Review the information on the *Visit Summary* tab to confirm that the correct codes are displaying.

10. Once the information is confirmed in the *Visit Summary* screen, on the *Visit Summary* screen place a check mark next to *Check out Patient?* (**Figure 6-15**), and click *Save*.

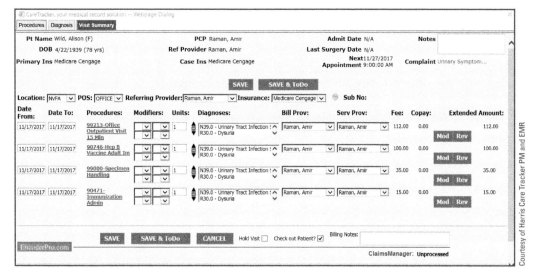

Figure 6-15   Alison Wild Visit Summary Screen

11. You must wait for the message "An error occurred connecting to Claims manager. Transaction saved" before moving on.

12. Click on the "OK" button.

13. When the visit information is saved, the icon in the *Visit* column changes to "Visit Complete." (**Note:** If you don't see the change, "Refresh" the *Open Encounters* screen to see the updated *Visit* column entry. You can refresh clicking on the *Refresh* icon located next to the *Provider* name field.

 Print a screenshot of the updated Open Encounters window, label it "Activity 6-3," and place it in your assignment folder.

14. You will sign the note in Activity 6-4. After both the progress note and billing process are complete, the encounter is deleted from the *Open Encounters* application and is saved under the *Encounter* section of the patient's medical record for reference. Harris CareTracker PM and EMR updates the status of the *Note* and *Visit* columns to "Complete," and "Visit Complete."

Activity 6-4
Sign and Print a Progress Note

The *Unsigned Notes* application displays a list of progress notes that are not signed or that require a co-signature by the provider set in the batch. A co-signature is required when a progress note is documented by a non-physician provider such as a physician assistant (PA) or a nurse practitioner (NP). Once again, acting as a clinical MA or provider, access the *Unsigned Notes* application (**Figure 6-16**) from one of the following locations:

- *Clinical Today* module > *Tasks* tab > *Unsigned Notes* (from the *Tasks* menu on the right side of the window) or click an unsigned notes task in the *All Tasks* window. You can sort on the *Tasks* column to easily identify unsigned note tasks. (**Note:** If the *Unsigned Note* is not displaying, change the provider to "All" and click the refresh icon.)

- An alternative method is to click the *Clinical Today* module, and then click *Unsigned Notes* from the *Quick Tasks* menu (on the right side of the window).

The *Unsigned Notes* application lists notes that the treating and supervising provider must review and sign. You can sign the note directly from the following locations:

- *Unsigned Notes* application

- *Progress Notes* application

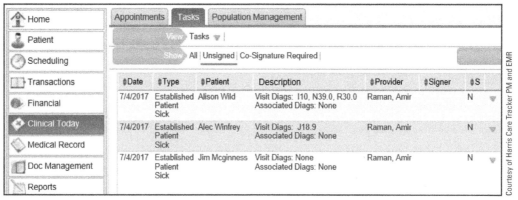

Figure 6-16   Unsigned Notes Application

It is important to know that once a progress note is signed, you can no longer make changes to it, and any open items/orders that were not completed prior to signing the note will not display within the A&P. Having confirmed that all tasks outlined in the A&P are completed, sign the note.

To Sign a Note:

Once you have confirmed that all tasks outlined in the A&P are completed:

1. Access the *Unsigned Notes* application by clicking on the *Home* module, *Open Encounters* under the *Clinical* column.

2. In the *Encounters* screen, *Note* column you will find Ms. Wild's note, stating "Not Signed."

3. Click on "Not Signed" in the *Note* column and the progress note launches. **Hint:** If you do not see the note, remember to change the "Resource" (Provider) to *All* and then search.

4. Review the progress note for accuracy then click the *Sign* 🖉 icon.

5. A message prompts to confirm the action (**Figure 6-17**). Click *OK*. (**Note:** Alternatively, you could point to the *Arrow* icon in the *Action* menu and click *Edit Note* to open the note in a new window, review, make changes, and sign or co-sign the note.)

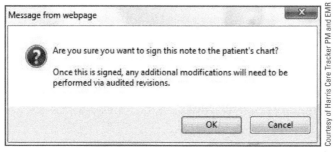

Figure 6-17   Sign Note Pop-Up Window

6. Once the *Progress Note* is signed, it will disappear from the *Unsigned Notes* application. **Note:** You may need to click the *Refresh* icon first.

7. With patient Alison Wild in context, click on the *Medical Record* module.

8. Click on *Progress Notes* from the *Patient Health History* pane, and select the progress note you created for Alison Wild. The note launches on the right side of the pane.

9. Click the *Print* icon on the *Progress Note* (**Figure 6-18**) you just signed. A dialog box will display where you can select *Print* or *PDF*. Select *Print*.

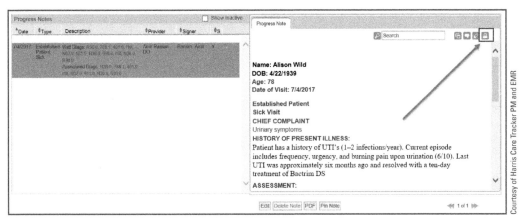

Figure 6-18   Progress Note with Print Icon

10. Close the dialog box when you have finished printing.

 Print the signed Progress Note. Label it "Activity 6-4," and place it in your assignment folder.

11. Now access the *Open Encounters* application again from the *Home* module > *Dashboard* tab > *Open Encounters* link (*Clinical* section). Using the drop-down feature next to *Provider*, select *All*, and then click the *Change Resource* (Click to Search) icon to refresh the screen. You will note that Alison Wild's encounter is no longer listed in the *Open Encounters* link.

CRITICAL THINKING At the beginning of this chapter, you were challenged to assess how information contained in the A&P of the progress note may affect your work as a billing/coding professional. The scenario presented listed various options to resolve the coding error. After completing this chapter and its activities, has your understanding changed? What approach would yield the best result for the practice, the flow of information, and a collaborative work environment? How does the accuracy of information contained in the EMR affect you as a billing/coding professional? Explain how you reached your conclusion.

CASE STUDIES

If the demographic pop-up alerts you to missing information when you pull the patient into context, it is best practice to update as necessary. Update patients' PCP, subscriber numbers, and confirm (Y) to Consent, HIE, and NPP as needed throughout the remainder of your activities and case studies.

(continues)

CASE STUDIES *(continued)*

Case Study 6-1

Repeat Activity 6-4 and sign and print the progress note for Jim Mcginness.
Note for future reference: Do you recall from Chapter 4 that when Mr. Mcginness was checked in for his visit his insurance information was not updated and that no copy of his current insurance card was scanned? Consider this as you proceed with billing and coding activities and think about what effect this may have on the revenue cycle.

You also note that Jim paid his former copay amount upon check-in ($35.00) and that his new insurance has only a $20.00 copay. Keep this in mind during later activities when addressing an overpayment.

Print the signed progress note and label it "Case Study 6-1." Place both documents in your assignment folder.

Case Study 6-2

Repeat Activity 6-4 and sign and print the progress note for Alec Winfrey.

Print the signed progress note, label it "Case Study 6-2," and place it in your assignment folder.

Case Study 6-3

Repeat Activity 6-2 and Capture the Visit for patient Harriet Oshea using the following CPT and ICD-10 codes (**Hint:** refer to the *History* tab in the *Scheduling* module to determine the date of Ms. Oshea's appointment).

In the *Procedures* tab, select CPT® codes 99213, 73565, 73520, and 36415 for this visit.

In the *Diagnosis* tab, select ICD-10 code M15.0.

After saving the Visit, print the Visit Summary screen, label it "Case Study 6-3," and place it in your assignment folder.

Case Study 6-4

Repeat Activity 6-4 and sign and print the progress note for Harriet Oshea (**Hint:** refer to the *History* tab in the *Scheduling* module to determine the date of Ms. Oshea's encounter date).

Print the signed progress note, label it "Case Study 6-4," and place it in your assignment folder.

Billing

7

Learning Objectives

1. Create a batch for financial transactions.
2. Manually enter a charge.
3. Edit an unposted charge.
4. Generate electronic and paper claims.
5. Perform activities related to electronic remittance including: posting payments and adjustments, and reconciling insurance payments.

Real-World Connection

Your challenge is to become familiar with the many different types of insurance plans and the effects on the practice when there is an issue regarding noncovered services. In order for the medical practice to be profitable, fees must be collected from patients for services rendered. The fees and copay can be collected at the time of the visit, or you can bill the patient after a claim has been submitted to the insurance company, depending on the type of insurance and the policy of the practice. It is NVFHA policy that copays must be collected from the patient at the office for each encounter. We only bill the copay when the patient does not have any form of payment available at the time of service. Upon receipt of payment from the insurance company and after any adjustment to the contracted rate is applied, the balance due will be billed to the patient.

Although it may be a delicate issue, you will be responsible for communicating the fees for services to patients. This discussion should take place prior to the patient's appointment with the physician to avoid an awkward situation, and again at any time there is a test ordered that will also include separate fees. With the ever-changing insurance environment and mandates from the Affordable Care Act (ACA), and the possible repeal and replacement of the ACA, you must verify the patient's insurance plan, deductibles, out-of-pocket amounts, and confirm that NVFHA is in fact contracted with the patient's insurance company before providing services. The deductibles with insurance plans available through the ACA and exchanges are extremely high (average for individuals is $6,500 per year or more and $10,000 or more per family). Consider how such a high deductible and out-of-pocket expenses will affect the patient's ability to pay and also the possibility that the patient may delay seeking health care due to the high insurance deductible.

If the patient's insurance is not contracted with NVFHA, the patient will be responsible for the entire fee. In some cases, patients will be forced to change providers to one that is contracted with their insurance; otherwise the costs would be unaffordable to the patient. Changing doctors is very stressful to many patients. Often they have developed relationships that span many years or decades. Therefore, it is important that you have an understanding of the various types of insurance and how to communicate effectively with patients in an articulate and compassionate manner. Even within the many types of insurance, copays and deductibles can vary widely. Some health plans have large deductibles and large copays. Other plans may require no copay at the time of visit, but the patient will pay a percentage of the contracted rate for the service.

Real-World Connection (continued)

When you register a new patient and collect patient demographic information over the phone, you will gather insurance information as well. This will help determine what type of fee or payment will be required of the patient, and confirm that our practice is contracted with the patient's insurance carrier. The office policy must be clearly stated to the patients on the telephone, by written communication (on forms the patient must complete and sign), and by way of posted notices in the waiting room. Patients should be gently reminded in a very professional manner that payment will be expected at the time of service. Our automated answering system also conveys fee and payment options available.

Before you begin the activities in this chapter, refresh your memory on working with Harris CareTracker by referring back to the Best Practices list on page xiv of this workbook. Following best practices will help you complete work quickly and accurately.

CREATE A BATCH

Learning Objective 1: Create a batch for financial transactions.

Activity 7-1

Create a Batch for Billing and Charges

Setting Operator Preferences

In order to perform any financial transactions, you must create a batch or have a batch open. Harris CareTracker PM will prompt you to create a batch unless you have already created a batch that has not yet been posted. You can view open batch(es) by clicking on the *Home* module > *Dashboard* tab > *Billing* header > *Open Batches* link (**Figure 7-1**). You begin by setting the operator preferences as completed in Chapter 4, Activity 4-3. Create a *Batch* as instructed to begin your activities in this chapter.

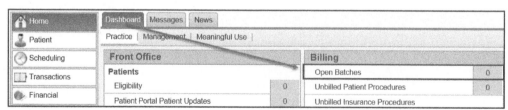

Figure 7-1   Open Batches Link   Courtesy of Harris CareTracker PM and EMR

Because you will have been working in various activities in more than one fiscal period, always work in the "current" fiscal period unless otherwise instructed (e.g., if you begin an activity in September, complete all the related activities in that period. If you start a new activity unrelated to a previous period [e.g., in December], you would then use the new period [December]). Although you will be instructed to complete activities and post batches, *never* close a period.

1. Prior to creating a batch, you will need to open the fiscal period for which you will be entering activities. Go to the *Administration* module > *Practice* tab > *System Administration, Financial* headers > *Open/Close Period* link (**Figure 7-2**).

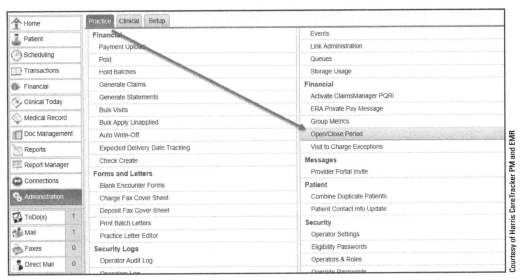

Figure 7-2   Open/Close Period Link

2. If the period is not already "Open", open the fiscal period for the activities you are posting. Use the fiscal period and month of Alison Wild's first appointment.

3. Click *Save* (**Figure 7-3**).

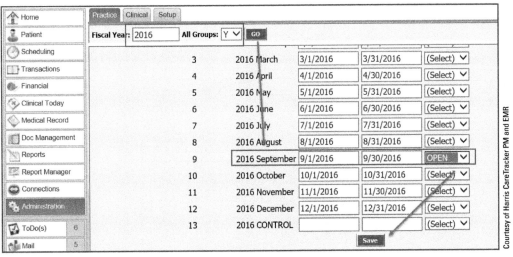

Figure 7-3   Open Fiscal Period for September 2016

4. Click the *Batch* ▌ icon on the *Name Bar* and the *Operator Encounter Batch Control* dialog box will display.

5. Then click *Edit.* (**Figure 7-4**).

6. Click *Create Batch.* The *Batch Master* dialog box displays (**Figure 7-5**).

7. Change the *Batch Name* to "Ch7Charges" (**Figure 7-6**). Do not use symbols when editing the name.

8. By default, the *Group Id* displays the name of your group.

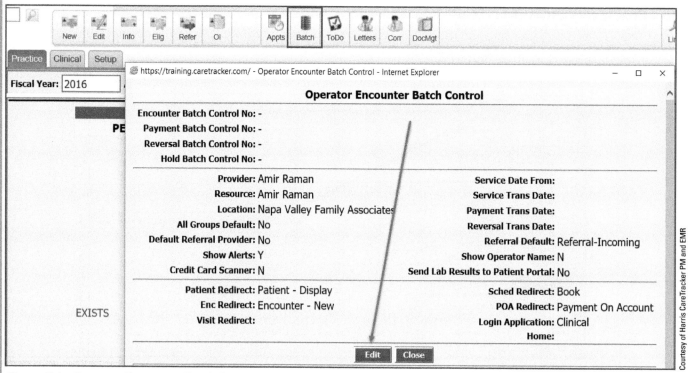

Figure 7-4   Operator Encounter Batch Control Dialog Box—Edit

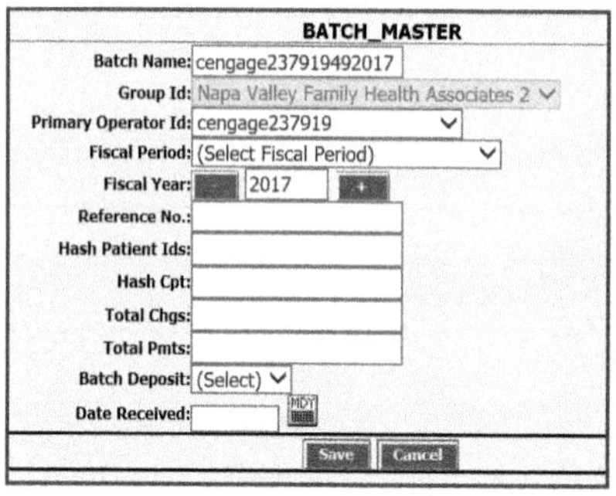

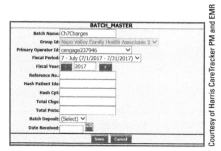

Figure 7-5   Batch Master Dialog Box

Figure 7-6   Change Batch Name

9. By default, the *Primary Operator Id* displays your user name. This cannot be changed.

10. By default, the *Fiscal Year* displays the current financial year set up for your company.

11. In the *Fiscal Period* list, click the period to post financial transactions. The list only displays fiscal periods that are currently open. Select the current fiscal period.

12. Leave the *Reference No*; *Hash Patient Ids*; *Hash Cpt*; *Total Chgs*; *Total Pmts*; and *Batch Deposit* fields blank.

13. In the *Date Received* box, enter the date the encounter was created in MM/DD/YYYY format or click the *calendar* 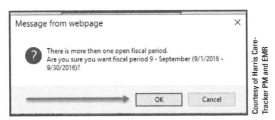 icon and select the date. Select the date of Alison Wild's first appointment.

14. Click *Save*. If you have more than one period open, a pop-up warning (**Figure 7-7**) will appear asking you to confirm the fiscal period. Click *OK*.

Figure 7-7   Fiscal Period Pop-Up Warning

15. Harris CareTracker PM and EMR displays the *Operator Encounter Batch Control* dialog box with the new batch information (**Figure 7-8**).

16. Further *Edit* your batch using the drop-down arrow next to each field and updating the provider, resource, location, and so on, if needed.

    a. If not already selected, select "Amir Raman" as the *Provider* and *Resource*.

    b. Change your *Login Application* to *Home*.

    c. Leave the *Home* field as *Practice*.

17. Click *Save*.

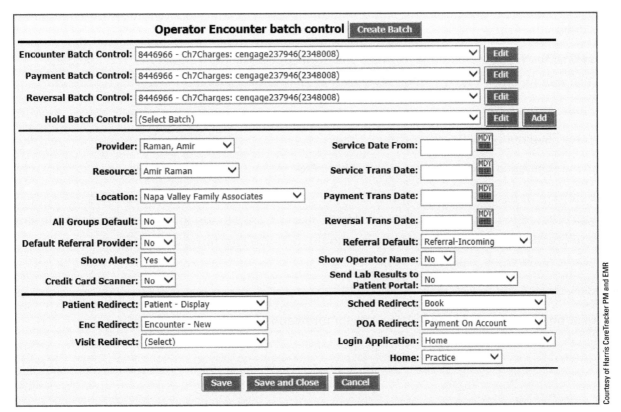

Figure 7-8   Ch7Charges Batch Information

18. Write down your "Encounter Batch Control No." for future reference (should include "Ch7Charges").

    _____.

 Print the Operator Encounter Batch Control screen, label it "Activity 7-1," and place it in your assignment folder.

19. Click the "X" in the upper-right corner to close the dialog box.

MANUALLY ENTER A CHARGE

Learning Objective 2: Manually enter a charge.

Activity 7-2
Posting a Patient Payment

Charges are financial transactions that require a batch to be created before entering and saving a charge. Having created your batch in Activity 7-1, complete Activity 7-2 to post a patient payment. Although Ms. Wild does not have a copay with her Medicare insurance, she knows that she will have an amount due after Medicare pays its portion. She does not like to owe money on her account, so at checkout, she would like to make a payment toward any balance that may be due.

1. Pull patient Alison Wild into context.

2. Open the *Transactions* module. The *Charge* application displays by default.

3. Click on the *Pmt on Acct* tab.

4. In Chapter 4, you learned how to enter and print copay receipts for patients. Following the instructions in Activity 4-5, enter a payment on account for patient Alison Wild.

5. Enter Amount: $25.00

6. Enter Payment Type "Payment-Patient Check."

7. In the Reference # field, enter check number "4434."

8. Enter the appointment date (*Trans. Date*) to be applied to Alison's payment (the appointment you created in Chapter 4). In the *Appt* field, use the drop down and select the appointment you created in Chapter 4. Your screen should look like **Figure 7-9**. (**Note:** Do not check the "Copay?" box.)

9. Click *Quick Save*.

10. Click on the *Receipts* tab and print a receipt for Alison Wild.

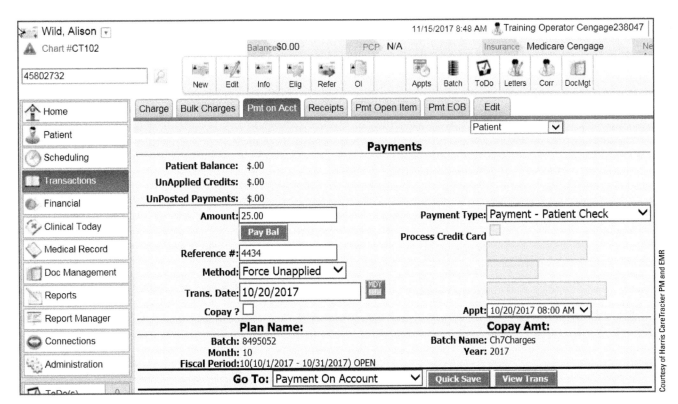

Figure 7-9   Alison Wild Payment on Account

 Print the receipt, label it "Activity 7-2," and place it in your assignment folder.

You will <u>not</u> post the batch at this time because you will complete additional activities before running a journal and posting a batch.

Activity 7-3
Manually Enter a Charge for a Patient

Having entered the payment on account for Alison Wild in Activity 7-2, continue your billing activities by manually entering a charge for a different patient not on the schedule.

1. Following the steps in Activity 7-1, create a new batch using today's current month and year. (**Note:** If the fiscal period and fiscal year are not already open, you will need to open them before creating the batch.) Set the batch parameters as follows:

   a. *Batch Name*: SmithSNF

   b. *Fiscal Year*: Use the current year

   c. *Fiscal Period*: Use the current month

   d. *Provider* and *Resource*: Raman, Amir

2. After the current fiscal period is open and you have the new batch created, pull patient Darryl Smith into context.

3. Open the *Transactions* module. The *Charge* application displays by default, displaying the charge screen. If the *Charge* application is not displaying, click on the *Charge* tab.

TIP You may get a pop-up stating "Please check Batch." If so, click *OK*. The *Operator Encounter Batch* screen will display. In the *Encounter Batch Control* field, you'll see that the "SmithSNF" batch you created is selected. Click "Save and Close."

4. Manually enter a "Skilled Nursing Facility" charge using the following charge-related information:

   a. Using the *Location* drop-down, select "NVSNF."

   b. Using the [Tab] key will automatically populate the *POS* with "SKILLED NURSING FACILITY."

   c. Enter *Ref Provider* "Dr. Raman."

FYI In the center of the screen, the *Visit* button will be grayed out (**Figure 7-10**). In a live application, clicking the *Visit* button allows you to access the *Visit* window in which CPT and ICD-10 codes can be selected for the patient.

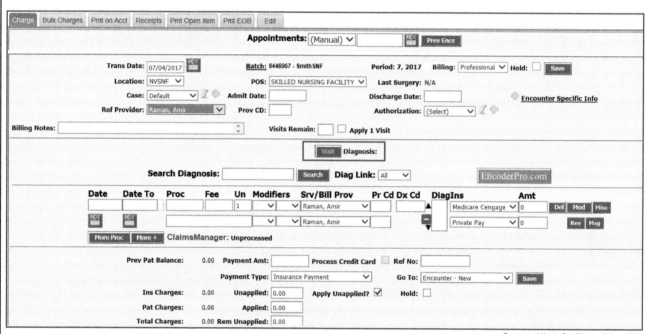

Figure 7-10   SNF Charge   Courtesy of Harris CareTracker PM and EMR

5. If there have been previous ICD codes entered for this patient, you can place a check mark by the desired code to select it. Select codes R07.89 (Other chest pain), I10, and I50.9. If any of these codes are not listed, type the code (e.g., "I10") in the *Search Diagnosis* field and then click *Search*. Harris CareTracker PM will pull in the diagnosis code in the *Diag* field (**Figure 7-11**). Repeat code searches as necessary until you have all the three codes are listed.

6. Click on *EncoderPro.com* to review the codes selected and determine if they are appropriate for the visit/charge. Click "X" to close the *EncoderPro* window.

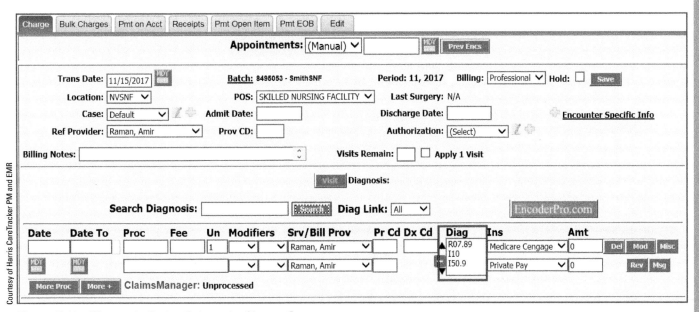

Figure 7-11   Diagnosis Codes Selected—Charge Screen

7. Enter today's date in the *Date* and *Date To* fields. A date can either be entered manually in MM/DD/YYYY format or can be selected from the *Calendar* 🔲 function. The date must be within the open period in your current batch.

8. Enter the code "99212" in the *Proc* field, and hit the [Tab] key. The procedure description, fee, and the amount to be charged to the patient's insurance and to the patient will be populated, and the *Modifiers* will become the active field. Do not select any modifiers.

9. Click on the *More Proc* button, which brings up another billing line. Enter CPT® code "G0180" in the *Proc* field. Hit the [Tab] key and the *Procedure Search* pop-up box will appear (**Figure 7-12**). Click on the code or description and the procedure will be pulled in to the charge box.

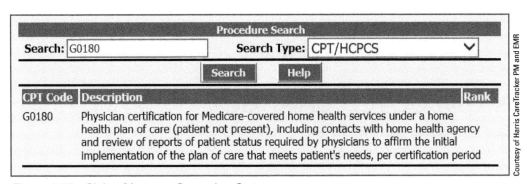

Figure 7-12   ClaimsManager Screening Status

10. Enter $100 in the *Fee* field because this CPT® code is not on the NVFHA fee schedule.

11. Select "Raman, Amir" from the *Srv/Bill Prov* drop-down list, if not already selected (**Figure 7-13**).

🖨 **Print the Charge Screen, label it "Activity 7-3," and place it in your assignment folder.**

12. Click *Save*. You will receive an error message (**Figure 7-14**) because your student version is not connected to *Claims Manager*. However, the transaction will be saved, and the patient is taken out of context. (**Note:** It may take a few moments for this task to save. You <u>must</u> wait until you receive the "error" message "Transaction Saved" before moving on.)

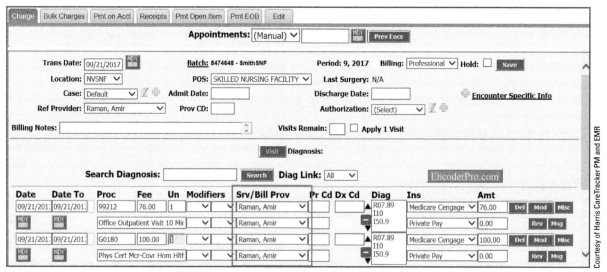

Figure 7-13   SNF Procedure (CPT) Codes in Charge Screen

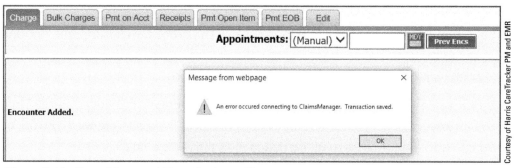

Figure 7-14   Error Message When Saving a Charge

13. Click *OK* and the patient is removed from context and "Encounter Added" displays on your screen.

14. Your manually entered charge is now saved.

EDIT AN UNPOSTED CHARGE

Learning Objective 3: Edit an unposted charge.

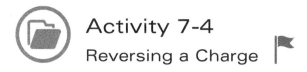

Activity 7-4
Reversing a Charge

Although it is not required to edit charges, there will be times when you will find it necessary to edit an unposted charge (e.g., a biller is reviewing a charge and sees that the incorrect CPT® code was assigned to the claim). Using the charge entered in Activity 7-3, edit the unposted charge.

1. Review the batch screen to confirm you are still working in the "SmithSNF" batch.

2. Pull patient Darryl Smith into context.

3. Click the *Transactions* module. Harris CareTracker PM and EMR opens the *Charge* application.

4. Click on the *Edit* tab. When *Edit* is clicked, all of the procedures entered in the patient's account along with each financial transaction linked to it will display (**Figure 7-15**) beginning with the most recent date of service. Locate the procedure that needs to be entirely reversed on the patient's account. (**Note:** You may need to scroll down the screen to locate the charge in question.) As a biller, you have noticed that CPT® code 99212 is incorrect, and want to change it to CPT® code 99214.

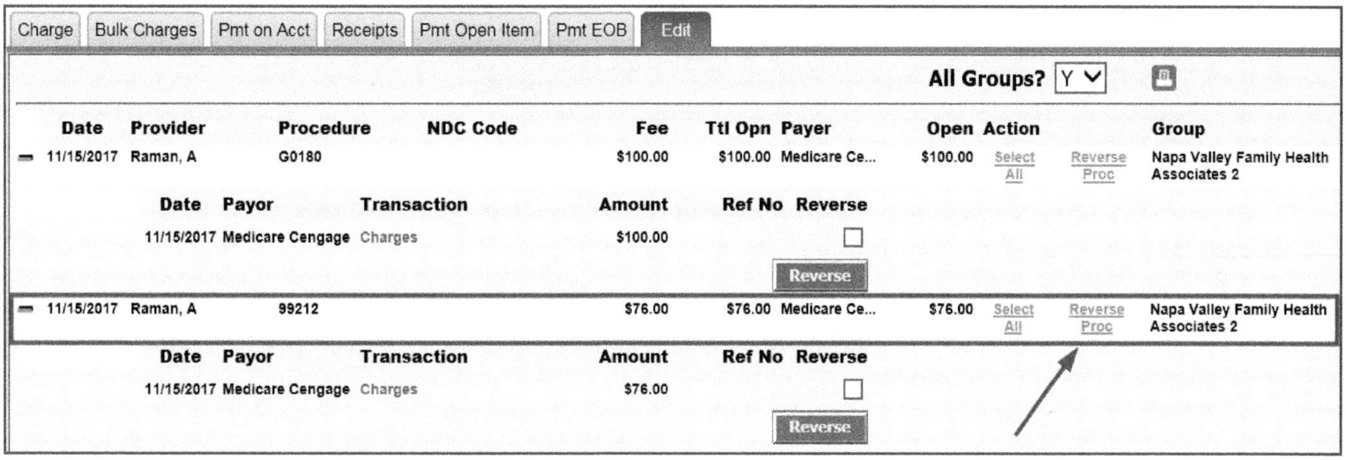

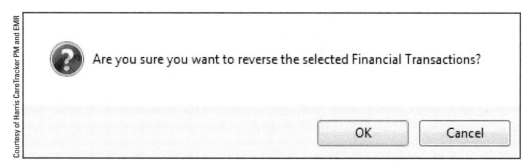

Figure 7-15   Edit Unposted Charge for Edith Robinson

5. Select the *Reverse Proc* link on the 99212 charge *only* (see Figure 7-15). (**Note**: If you click on the *Reverse* button, all of the selected transactions are reversed. Do *not* click on the *Reverse* button)

6. You will receive a pop-up warning message (**Figure 7-16**) asking "Are you sure you want to reverse the selected Financial Transactions?" Click *OK*. The transaction will be reversed (see **Figure 7-17**). (**Note:** If you receive the error message "The Reversal Date must be within Period Start and End Dates: xx/xx/20xx and: xx/xx/20xx," it may be due to a "compatibility" issue with your browser. Refer to Best Practices regarding compatibility.)

Figure 7-16   Reverse Financial Transaction Warning

🖳 **Print the Edit Unposted Charge screen, label it "Activity 7-4a," and place it in your assignment folder.**

| Charge | Bulk Charges | Pmt on Acct | Receipts | Pmt Open Item | Pmt EOB | Edit |

Date	Provider	Procedure	NDC Code	Fee	Ttl Opn	Payer	Open	Action		Group
11/15/2017	Raman, A	G0180		$100.00	$100.00	Medicare Ce...	$100.00	Select All	Reverse Proc	Napa Valley Family Health Associates 2

	Date	Payor	Transaction	Amount	Ref No	Reverse
	11/15/2017	Medicare Cengage	Charges	$100.00		☐

Reverse

Date	Provider	Procedure			Fee	Ttl Opn	Payer	Open	Action		Group
11/15/2017	Raman, A	99212			$76.00	0.00	Medicare Ce...	0.00	Select All	Reverse Proc	Napa Valley Family Health Associates 2

	Date	Payor	Transaction	Amount	Ref No	Reverse
	11/15/2017	Medicare Cengage	Charges	$76.00		☐
	11/15/2017	Medicare Cengage	Charges	($76.00)		☐

Reverse

Figure 7-17   Reversed Charge

Courtesy of Harris CareTracker PM and EMR

7. Click back on the *Charge* tab in the *Transactions* module and complete the charge screen:

   a. *Location*: NVSNF

   b. *POS*: SKILLED NURSING FACILITY

   c. *Ref Provider*: Raman, Amir

   d. *Diagnosis*: R07.89, I10, I50.9

   e. *Date* and *Date To*: Use today's date

   f. Enter "99214" in the *Proc* field, and hit the [Tab] key. $245 should populate in the *Fee* field. If not, enter $245 into the *Fee* field.

🖨 **Print the Charge screen, label it "Activity 7-4b," and place it in your assignment folder.**

8. Click on *Save* to save the charge. ***Important!!*** Be sure to wait for the message "An error occurred connecting to ClaimsManager. Transaction saved" before moving forward.

9. Click *OK*, and your transaction is saved.

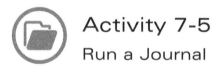

Activity 7-5
Run a Journal

Now that you have manually entered and edited unposted charges, the common workflow would be to complete the process by running a journal and posting your batch.

When you have finished entering data into your batch, you will run a journal to verify your batch and entry information. It is best practice to run a journal (as in Activity 4-18) prior to posting your batch to verify that you have entered all the financial transactions correctly in Harris CareTracker PM.

1. Go to the *Reports* module > *Reports* tab > *Financial Reports* header > *Todays Journals* link (**Figure 7-18**).

2. Harris CareTracker PM displays the *Todays Journal Options* screen. All of your group's open batches are listed in the *Todays Batches* box. You may need to click on the [+] sign to expand the *Batches* field (see **Figure 7-19**).

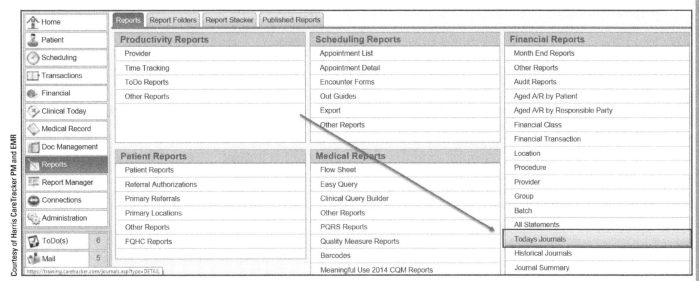

Figure 7-18   Todays Journals Link

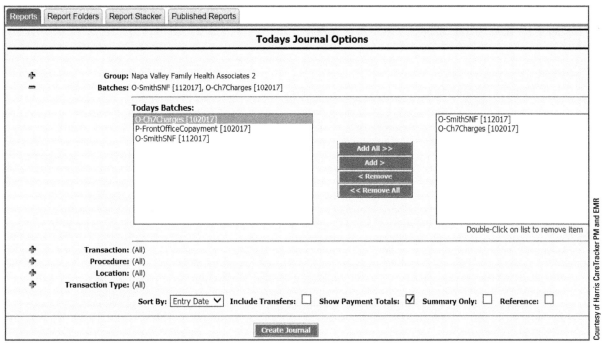

Figure 7-19   Expand Journal Batch Options

3. Select a batch to include in the journal either by double-clicking on the batch name or by clicking on the batch and then clicking *Add >*. Harris CareTracker PM adds the selected batches to the box on the right. Select and add batches "Ch7Charges" and "SmithSNF."

4. Scroll down to the bottom of the screen. From the *Sort By* drop-down list, select *Entry Date* (**Figure 7-20**).

5. Select the *Show Payment Totals* checkbox.

6. Click *Create Journal*. Harris CareTracker PM generates the journal (**Figure 7-21**).

7. To print, right-click on the journal and select *Print* from the shortcut menu.

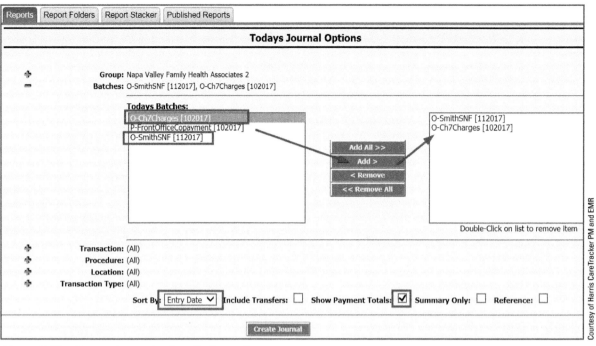

Figure 7-20   Create Journal—Sort By Entry Date

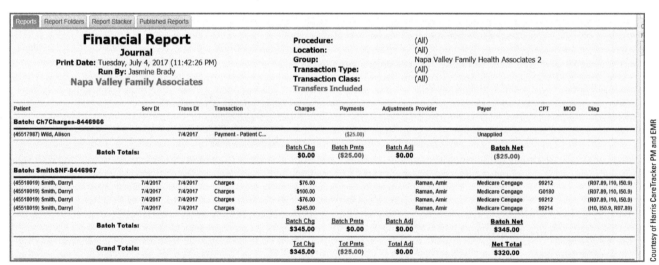

Figure 7-21   Journal—Financial Report

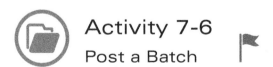 **Print the Journal, label it "Activity 7-5," and place it in your assignment folder.**

8. Close out of the *Journal* report by clicking back on the *Reports* module.

Activity 7-6
Post a Batch

Having balanced the money in your journal, post an open batch as directed in Activity 7-6 using the alternate method of posting batches outlined in the steps following:

1. Go to the *Administration* module > *Practice* tab > *Daily Administration* section > *Financial* header > *Post* link (**Figure 7-22**). Harris CareTracker PM displays a list of all open batches for the group.

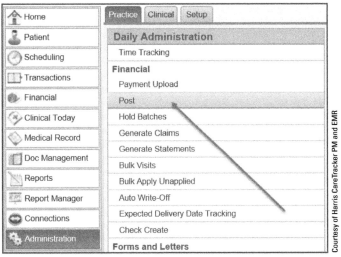

Figure 7-22   Post Link from Practice Tab

2. Check the box next to the batch(es) you want to post. Select *only* the batch "Ch7Charges" (**Figure 7-23**). Do *not* select or post the "SmithSNF" batch at this time.

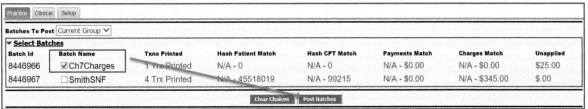

Figure 7-23   Post Batches   Courtesy of Harris CareTracker PM and EMR

 Print the Post Batches screen, label it "Activity 7-6," and place it in your assignment folder

3. Then click *Post Batches.*

BUILD AND GENERATE CLAIMS

Learning Objective 4: Generate electronic and paper claims.

Activity 7-7
Workflow for Electronic Submission of Claims

Harris CareTracker PM transmits electronic claims directly to insurance companies and to clearinghouses.

Claims can only be generated after your batch has been posted. You will simulate generating claims by following the steps in Activity 7-7. Because the *ClaimsManager* feature is not active in your student version of Harris CareTracker PM, the claim will not actually generate, but you will be able to complete the steps.

1. Go to the *Administration* module > *Practice* tab > *Daily Administration* section > *Financial* header > *Generate Claims* link (**Figure 7-24**). Harris CareTracker PM launches the *Generate Claims* application.

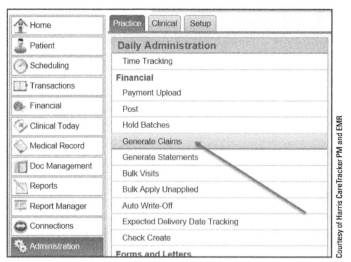

Figure 7-24   Generate Claims Link

2. Click *Generate Claims For This Group* (**Figure 7-25**). You may receive an error message stating "Error Queuing Claims" or a message saying "Claims are being Generated…" (**Figure 7-26**) because the *ClaimsManager* feature of your student version is not active. In a live environment, your screen would look like **Figure 7-27**, which states "Claims are Queued for all Groups under this Parent Company."

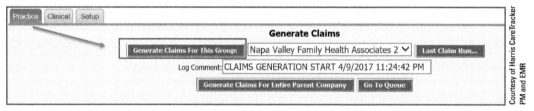

Figure 7-25   Generate Claims For This Group

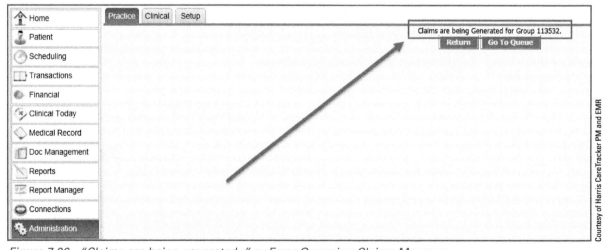

Figure 7-26   "Claims are being generated…" or Error Queueing Claims Message

3. Whether or not you have received an error message, click on *Go to Queue* and a report will generate (**Figure 7-28**). **Figure 7-29** represents an example of the *Claims Queue* in a live environment, which displays the *Claims Worklist*. Since you are working in a student environment, all of your queues will be empty.

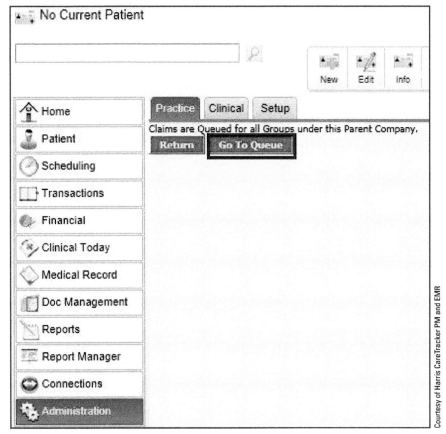

Figure 7-27   Claims Generated

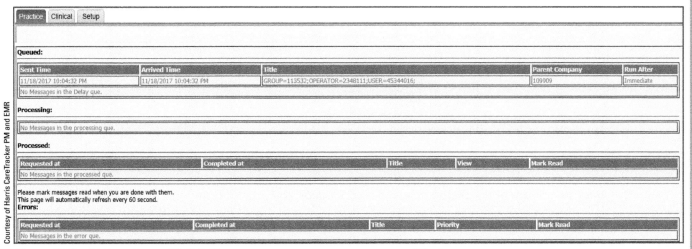

*Figure 7-28   Claims Queue (**NOTE**: The messages on your screen may differ.)*

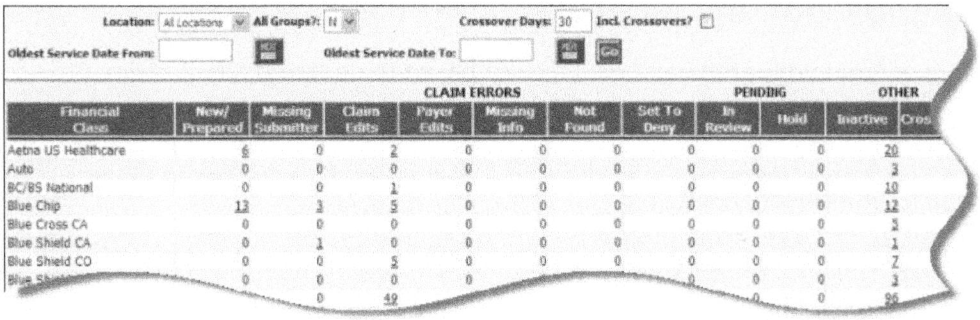

Figure 7-29   Claims Worklist

Print the Claims Queue window, label it "Activity 7-7," and place it in your assignment folder.

4. Click back on the *Administration* module to exit the claims queue. (**Note:** Claims wait in *Queue* to be processed at 5 p.m.)

Activity 7-8
Apply Settings to Print Paper Claims

Paper Claim Batches

Although paper claims are rare, there are occasions when you will need to submit one. In Harris CareTracker PM, paper claims are generated by way of the method outlined in Activity 7-9. To print paper claims, you must first apply print settings, as in Activity 7-8.

There are two ways to apply print settings in Harris CareTracker. For this activity, use the Harris CareTracker *Dashboard*.

1. Go to the *Home* module > *Dashboard* tab > *Billing* section > *Unprinted Paper Claim Batches* link. The application displays the *Print Options* window.

2. Click the *Print Options* button in the upper-right corner of the screen.

3. Locate the desired claim form ("1500 CMS Paper Form") in the list and then enter the margin size for the form in the corresponding *Offset Top* field (enter "10") and *Offset Left* field (enter "10") if not already populated (**Figure 7-30**).

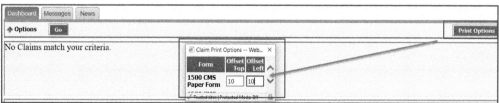

Figure 7-30   *Apply Settings to Print Paper Claims*   Courtesy of Harris CareTracker PM and EMR

 Print the Claim Print Options window, label it "Activity 7-8," and place it in your assignment folder.

4. Scroll to the bottom of the dialog box and click *Update*. You must log out and then log back in to Harris CareTracker PM and EMR before the setting takes effect.

Activity 7-9
Build and Generate a Paper Claim

Now that you have entered your print settings, you will be set to generate paper claims.

Patient Darryl Smith

1. Pull patient Darryl Smith into context.

2. Click the *OI▊* tab in the *Name* bar.

3. Click on *Instant Claim* in the *First Clm* column (**Figure 7-31**) for Procedure code 99214. Harris CareTracker PM displays the *Claims Summary* in the lower frame of the screen.

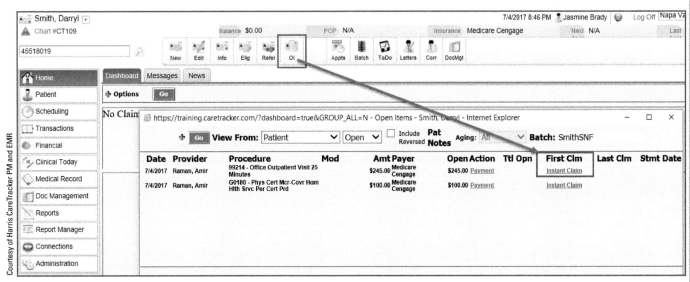

Figure 7-31   First Clm Column—Darryl Smith

4. Place a check mark in the rows for Procedure codes 99214 and G0180. Do <u>not</u> place a check mark in the row for Procedure code 99212.

5. Then click *Build Claim.* You will now note that the date you performed the activity is listed in the *First Clm* column.

6. Click on the date in the *First Clm* column for Procedure 99214 (**Figure 7-32**). Harris CareTracker PM displays the *Claims Summary* in the lower frame of the screen.

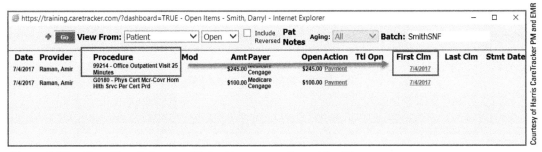

Figure 7-32   First Clm Column—Claim Summary; Darryl Smith

📑 **Print the Claims Summary window, label it "Activity 7-9A," and place it in your assignment folder.**

7. Scroll down and click the *Rebill To= = >* drop-down list at the bottom of the screen and select *Paper 1500*. Click *Rebuild Paper*. Because this is a simulated activity you will receive an error message (see **Figure 7-33**).

8. Close out of the error message and then close out of the *Open Items* screen by clicking on "X."

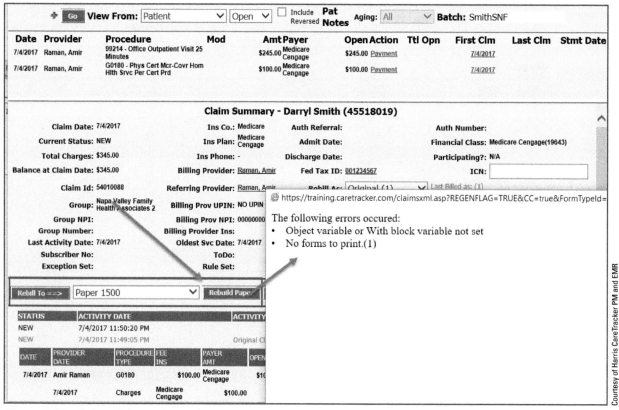

Figure 7-33   Select Rebuild Paper Claim—Paper Claim Error Message

FYI In a live environment, Harris CareTracker PM would have generated the HCFA 1500 CMS Paper Form (**Figure 7-34**). To print the form, you would right-click on the form and select Print from the shortcut menu. **Figures 7-35** and **7-36** provide examples of the HCFA and Workers Comp HCFA forms.

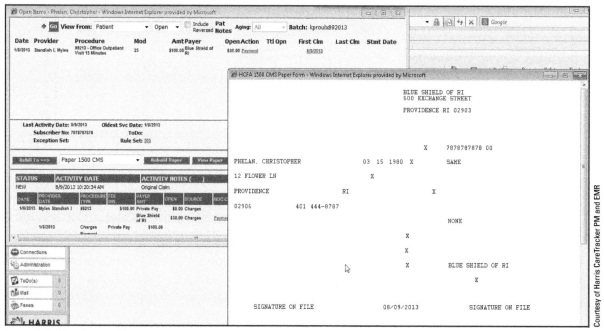

Figure 7-34   Paper Claim to 1500

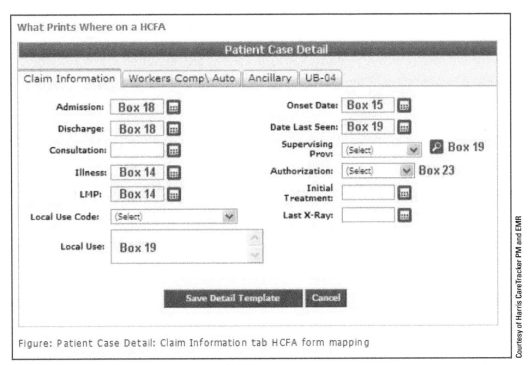

Figure: Patient Case Detail: Claim Information tab HCFA form mapping

Figure 7-35   What Prints Where on an HCFA

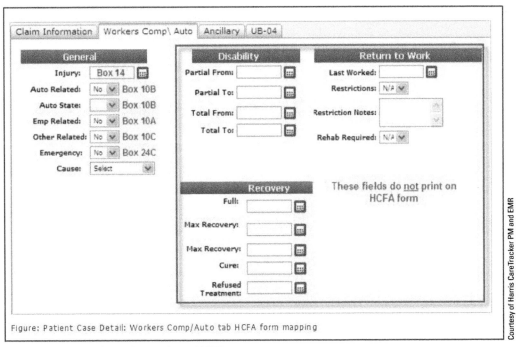

Figure: Patient Case Detail: Workers Comp/Auto tab HCFA form mapping

Figure 7-36   Workers Comp/Auto HCFA

ELECTRONIC REMITTANCE

Learning Objective 5: Perform activities related to electronic remittance including: posting payments and adjustments, and reconciling insurance payments.

Activity 7-10

Save Charges; Process a Remittance

Remittances received electronically in Harris CareTracker PM are identified in the *Electronic Remittances* application in the *Billing* section of the *Dashboard* (**Figure 7-37**). Harris CareTracker PM matches the transactions on the electronic remittance to a specific patient, date of service, CPT® code, and charge amount.

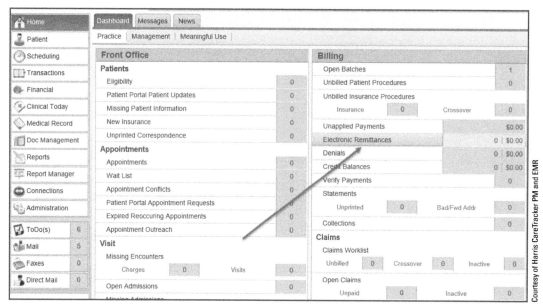

Figure 7-37   Electronic Remittances Link

There is a normal flow of payment activity in Harris CareTracker PM that begins when a patient pays his or her copayment. Copayments are entered in Harris CareTracker PM when the patient checks in or checks out (depending on the office workflow). Next, a claim is sent to the insurance company after the patient visit. In Harris CareTracker PM, most claims are transmitted electronically; however, paper forms are sometimes mailed. When bills are transmitted electronically, the payment is received electronically or on a paper EOB/RA.

Open Items is an application in the *Financial* module. There is an identical application accessed via the *Pmt Open Item* tab in the *Transactions* module, and this application can also be accessed as a window by clicking the *OI* 🔲 button on the *Name Bar*. The *Open Items* application is used to view all dates of service and the associated procedures, financial transactions, and claims activity (**Figure 7-38**). In this application, you can enter many different types of financial transactions including patient payments, insurance

Figure 7-38   Open Items

Courtesy of Harris CareTracker PM and EMR

payments, third-party payments, transfer balances, refunds, and apply unapplied money. You can also view the procedure details of each procedure, enter denial descriptions, attach statement messages to appear on patient statements, view a claim history, potentially rebill a claim, view electronic responses received from insurance companies, and view EOB/RAs attached to payments.

> **TIP** You can access *Open Items* any of the following ways:
> - Left-click on an appointment in the *Book* application and select *Open Items*.
> - Click the *OI* button on the *Name Bar*.
> - Click the *Pmt Open Item* tab in the *Transactions* module. If you receive an error message that the batch in not open, click on the *Batch* icon in the *Name Bar*. The "SmithSNF" batch will display. Click *Edit*, then click *Save*. Click back on the *Transactions* module and the *Pmt Open Item* tab, and the *Open Item*(s) will display.

The total number and sum of remittances received electronically into Harris CareTracker PM displays on the *Dashboard* and a list of the received remittances that need to be posted into the system is accessed by clicking on the *Electronic Remittances* link. Electronic remittances should only be posted after the check (or electronic payment) is received from the insurance company.

Before posting payments via *Electronic Remittances*, select one patient from the remittance, pull the patient into context, click the *OI* button on the *Name Bar,* and verify that the date of service is still open in Harris CareTracker PM (**Figure 7-39**).

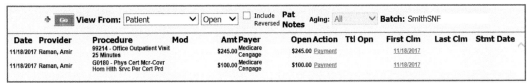

Figure 7-39   OI Electronic Remittance   Courtesy of Harris CareTracker PM and EMR

(A) Patient Alison Wild

1. Before you begin this activity, pull Alison Wild into context and refer back to Ms. Wild's encounter from Activity 4-1. (**Hint:** refer to the *Scheduling* module, *History* tab to locate the appointment date.) Record the date of the encounter for this activity: _____

2. Create a new batch and name it "7-10PostRAs." Use today's date for the *Fiscal Period* and *Fiscal Year*.

3. Update the *Provider* and *Resource* to Alison Wild's provider and PCP.

4. Click *Save and Close* on the newly created batch. If you receive a message that the "Service Date From is before today. Are you sure you want to save?", click *OK*.

5. Go to the *Home* module > *Dashboard* tab > *Visit* header > *Missing Encounters* > *Charges* link (**Figure 7-40**).

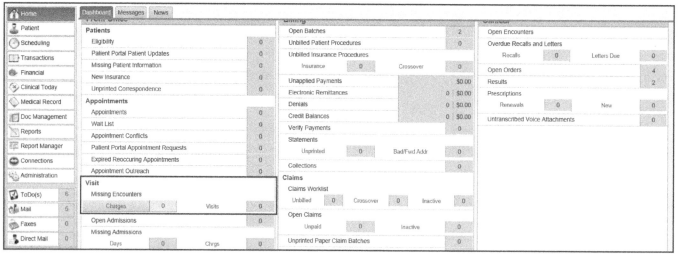

Figure 7-40   Missing Encounters/Charges Link

Courtesy of Harris CareTracker PM and EMR

6. Set the fields as follows:

    *   Change the beginning date to January 1 of the current year and change the ending date to today's date. (**Note**: By default, the ending date is yesterday and will not contain any entries made on the current date unless you change the ending date to today's date.) Be sure the dates include the date of the patient encounter from Activity 4-1.

    *   Select *All providers*.

    *   Select *All locations*.

    *   Select *Visits Yes*.

    *   Select *Charges No*.

7. Then click *Go* (**Figure 7-41**). You will see the *Charges* that have not been saved (**Figure 7-42**). If multiple patients have appointments on the same date, you will notice that the *Visits* and *Charges* buttons only appear in the row for the first patient with an appointment on that date. This is because when you are working in *OI*, if more than one charge (e.g., multiple patient visits) appears on the same date, *Charges* are saved for all patients with appointments on that date (see **Figure 7-43**).

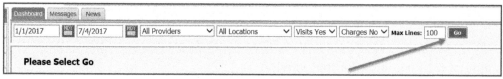

Figure 7-41   Visits Yes/Charges No

Courtesy of Harris CareTracker PM and EMR

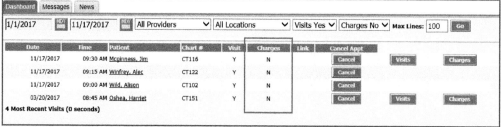

Figure 7-42   Charges Not Saved

Courtesy of Harris CareTracker PM and EMR

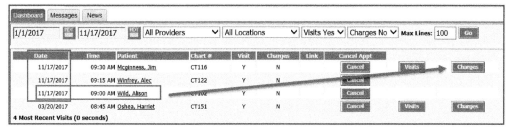

Figure 7-43   Visits and Charges Buttons

Courtesy of Harris CareTracker PM and EMR

8. In the *Date* column, locate the visit date (Figure 7-43) for patient Alison Wild's appointment from Activity 4-1. Then click on the *Charges* button on the right side of your screen for the date of service corresponding to her Activity 4-1 appointment. (Remember, the *Charges* button may not necessarily appear in Alison Wild's row; it may appear in the row of a different patient who has the same date of service as her.)

9. Now, click *Go* on the left side of your screen. The charges for all patient encounters on the Date of Service (DOS) display. **Note:** You may receive a pop-up message that says "Transaction Date must be within Period Start and End Dates: (of the date of your batch)." Click *OK* and the charges appear in the lower portion of your screen.

10. Since all the patients with charges display in the lower screen, you may need to scroll down to locate and review the charges for patient Alison Wild. We will assume here that the charges look okay.

11. Now, scroll down further to the bottom of the lower screen and click *Save* on the bottom left of your screen (**Figure 7-44**). (**Note:** If more than one charge [e.g., multiple patient visits] appear on the date, the *Charges* will be saved for all patients.)

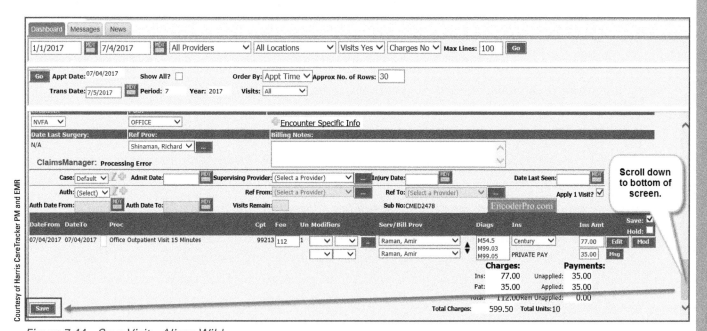

Figure 7-44   Save Visit—Alison Wild

Courtesy of Harris CareTracker PM and EMR

12. **Important!!** Wait until the "Transaction Saved" message appears before moving on. Then click *OK*. You will receive another pop-up stating "Bulk Charges Saved." Click *OK*.

13. With patient Alison Wild in context, click on the *OI* ⧠ button in the *Name Bar*. All captured charges for Ms. Wild's Activity 4-1 appointment now display.

14. Click on *Instant Claim* in the *First Clm* column.

15. Place a checkmark next to all of the charges.

16. Click *Build Claim.* The *Open Items* dialog box will now display with a date in the *First Clm* column.

17. Click on the *Payment* link in the *Action* column next to Procedure 99213. Harris CareTracker PM displays the payment window in the lower frame of the screen (**Figure 7-45**).

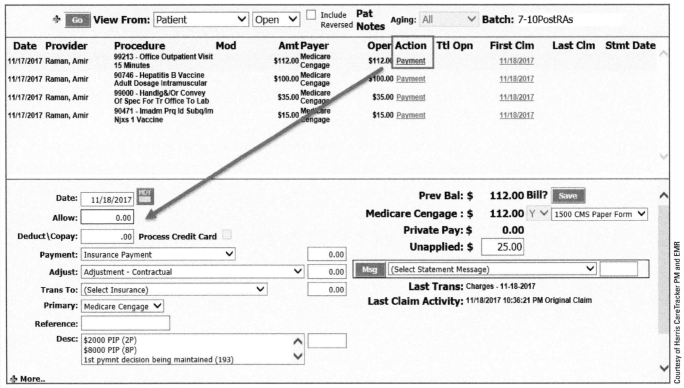

Figure 7-45   Payment Window in OI

18. In the payment window on the lower part of the screen, enter the information from Alison Wild's EOB/RA (Source Document 7-1, found at the end of this activity). Note, you will repeat this step for each of the Procedures on the EOB/RA. Your completed screen should look like **Figure 7-46**.

   a. *Date:* Use today's date, the date you "received the EOB/RA" for the appointment you created in Activity 4-1.

   b. *Allow:* Enter the information from the *Amount Allowed* column on the EOB/RA (Source Document 7-1). Now hit the [Tab] button on your keyboard.

   c. *Deduct/Copay:* Enter the information from the *Deduct/Coins/Copay* column on the EOB/RA (Source Document 7-1). Now hit the [Tab] button and this will populate the amount in the *Adjust* and *Transfer To* fields based on the information entered in the *Demographics* screen.

   d. *Payment:* Confirm that *Insurance Payment* is selected.

   e. *Adjust:* Confirm that *Adjustment—Contractual* is selected.

   f. *Trans To:* Confirm that *Private Pay* is selected.

   g. *Primary:* Confirm that *Medicare Cengage* is selected.

   h. *Reference:* Leave blank.

i. *Desc:* Enter "45" in the blank box to the right of the *Desc* field, and hit the [Tab] key.

j. *Msg:* Enter "CO" in the blank box to the right of the drop-down menu and hit the *[Tab]* key.

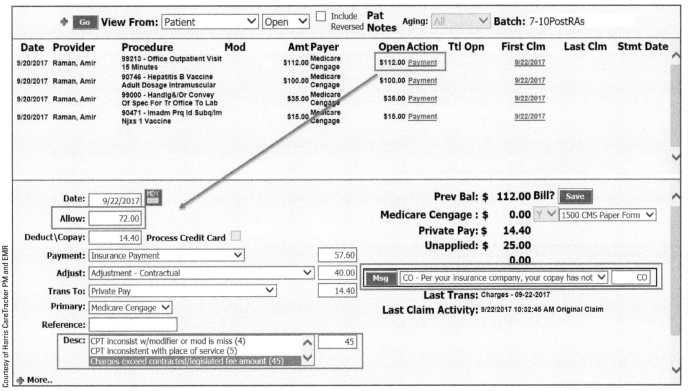

Figure 7-46   *Remittance Information in Payment Window*

📠 **Print the Process Remittance (OI screen), label it "Activity 7-10a," and place it in your assignment folder.**

19. Once you have entered the EOB/RA information for the *Payment*, click *Save.* Your transaction will be saved and the claim disappears.

20. Enter the information for each of the remaining procedures in Alison's EOB/RA. Because codes 90746 and 90471 are covered charges, you can use steps 17 through 19 as guidance to complete the information. Code 99000 is a charge that is not covered, and you will therefore need to use slightly different steps. You can tell this code is not covered because the full amount of the charge is listed in the "Not Covered (DENIAL)" column of the EOB/RA. Use the steps in the following Tip box to enter this not covered charge (denial).

 TIP

1. To enter a charge that is not covered (denial), follow the steps below. Note that you can tell what charges are not covered by checking the "Not Covered (DENIAL)" column to see if the full dollar amount of the charge is listed there.

2. **Note:** Be sure to use the [Tab] key so that fields automatically populate.

    a. *Date*: Enter today's date (within the *Fiscal Period/Fiscal Year* set in your batch).

    b. *Allow*: Leave blank (0.00).

(*continues*)

(*continued*)

    c. *Deduct/Copay:* Leave blank (0.00).

    d. *Payment*: Using the drop-down, select "Insurance Payment." **Note:** You may need to change the field first to (Select Payment Type) and then back to "Insurance Payment." Be sure you use the [Tab] key so that amounts will populate in the proper fields.

    e. *Adjust*: Select (Select Adjustment); enter "0.00." Make sure this field is "0.00." If you need to enter "0.00," be sure you use the [Tab] key so that amounts will populate in the proper fields.

    f. *Transfer To*: Use the drop-down and select *Private Pay*. This will automatically populate the amount field to the right of *Trans To*, as well as the *Prev Bal* and *Private Pay* fields.

    g. *Primary*: Leave blank (or it can remain "Medicare Cengage").

    h. *Reference*: Leave blank.

    i. *Desc*: Type "96" in the blank box to the right of *Desc* and hit [Tab]. This will select "Non-Covered charge (96)."

    j. In the *Msg* field, use the drop-down list and select *SEE BILLING NOTE*.

    k. Then click *Save*.

21. Continue entering the remaining payment information from the EOB/RA. When finished with all EOB/RA entries, close out of the *Open Items* window by clicking the "X" in the upper-right corner of the window.

22. Run a *Journal* for batch "7-10PostRAs."

    📠 **Print the Journal, label it "Activity 7-10A," and place in your assignment folder.**

(B) Patient Jim Mcginness

1. Process the Blue Shield Cengage remittance (EOB/RA) for his encounter using Source Document 7-2. If needed, refer to steps 13 through 19 of this activity above for information about how to process a remittance. (**Hint**: Note that if Jim's appointment was on a different date than Alison's, you will need to save his charges [refer to steps 5 through 12 of this activity for guidance] before you can process the remittance. If his appointment was on the same date as Alison's, then his charges have already been saved and you can proceed with processing the remittance.)

2. Upon completion, run a journal and review.

3. **Do not** post the "7-10PostRAs" batch at this time.

    📠 **Print the Journal, label it "Activity 7-10B," and place it in your assignment folder.**

You will note the Mr. Mcginness now has a credit balance. You recall in Chapter 4 when he checked in that his insurance information was not updated.

Source Document 7-1   Explanation of Benefits/Remittance Advice

MEDICARE CENGAGE

Medicare Cengage
P.O. Box 234434
San Francisco, CA 94137

Date: MM/DD/YYYY (Appt. date used in Activity 4-1)
Payment Number: 1334557
Payment Amount: $ 97.60

AMIR RAMAN, D.O.
Napa Valley Family Health Associates (NVFHA)
101 Vine Street
Napa, CA 94558

Account Number	Patient Name				Subscriber Number		Claim Number			
Dates of Service	Description of Service	Amount Charged	Not Covered (DENIAL)	Prov Adj Discount	Amount Allowed	Deduct/ Coins/ Copay	Paid to Provider	Adj Reason Code	Rmk Code	Patient Resp
CARE1357	Wild, Alison									
(Appt. date used in Activity 4-1)	99213	$112.00		$ 40.00	$ 72.00	$14.40	$57.60	45*		$14.40
(Appt. date used in Activity 4-1)	99000	$ 35.00	$35.00	$ 0.00	$ 0.00	$ 0.00	$35.00	96*		$35.00
(Appt. date used in Activity 4-1)	90746	$100.00		$ 60.00	$ 40.00	$ 8.00	$32.00	45*		$ 8.00
(Appt. date used in Activity 4-1)	90471	$ 15.00		$ 5.00	$ 10.00	$ 2.00	$ 8.00	45*		$ 2.00
TOTALS		$262.00	$35.00	$105.00	$157.00	$24.40	$132.60	$180.00		$59.40

Amount Allowed (45*) = Charges exceed your contracted/legislated fee arrangement
Amount Allowed (96*) = Not a covered code

Current Procedural Terminology (C) 2016 American Medical Association

Source Document 7-2   Explanation of Benefits/Remittance Advice

BLUE CROSS BLUE SHIELD - CENGAGE

Blue Shield – Cengage
PO Box 32245
Los Angeles, CA 90002

AMIR RAMAN, D.O.
Napa Valley Family Health Associates (NVFHA)
101 Vine Street
Napa, CA 94558

Date: MM/DD/YYYY (Appt. date used in Activity 4-1)
Payment Number: 6444578
Payment Amount: $ 80.00

Account Number	Patient Name					Subscriber Number		Claim Number			
Dates of Service	Description of Service	Amount Charged	Not Covered (DENIAL)	Prov Adj Discount	Amount Allowed	Deduct/ Coins/ Copay	Paid to Provider	Adj Reason Code	Rmk Code	Patient Resp
BCBS987	**Mcginness, Jim**									
(Appt. date used in Activity 4-1)	99213	$112.00		$12.00	$ 100.00	$20.00	$80.00	45*		$20.00
TOTALS		**$112.00**		**$12.00**	**$100.00**	**$20.00**	**$80.00**			**$20.00**

Amount Allowed (45*) = Charges exceed your contracted/legislated fee arrangement
Amount Allowed (20*) = Not a covered code

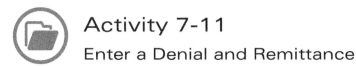

Activity 7-11

Enter a Denial and Remittance

Denials are claims that an insurance company has determined it will not pay, such as when a patient has not met his or her deductible. By working your denials separately from posting payments, you will improve the workflow and efficiency in your practice. Your student version of Harris CareTracker PM will not post *Denials* in your *Dashboard* because *ClaimsManager* is not active. The *Denials* screen can be accessed by going to the *Home* module > *Dashboard* tab > *Billing* header > *Denials* link (**Figure 7-47**).

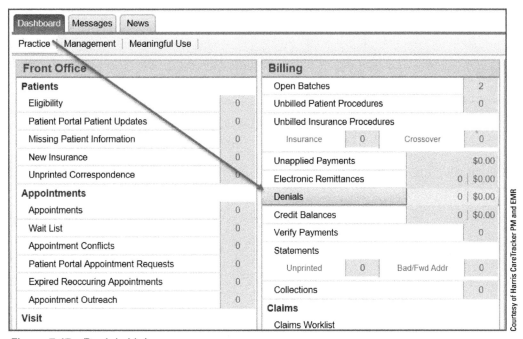

Figure 7-47   Denials Link

Using patient Darryl Smith, you will now post a denial and additional remittance to his account.

1. Before beginning this activity, click on *Batch* in the *Name Bar* and confirm you are still working in the "7-10PostRAs" batch.

2. With patient Darryl Smith in context, click on the *OI* button on the *Name Bar*.

3. You will see the charges for Mr. Smith's *Open Items*. You are going to now work the SNF edited charges for Procedure codes 99214 and G0180.

TIP

1. **Important!!** Only if you do <u>not</u> see the edited SNF charge for Procedure codes 99214 and G0180 in *OI*, go to the *Home* module > *Dashboard* tab > *Visit* header > *Missing Encounters/Visit* link and you will see that the *Charge* has not been saved.

To save the *Charges*, set the fields as follows:

*   Include the date of the patient encounter/manual charge.
*   Select *All providers*.

(continues)

(continued)

- Select *All locations.*
- Select *Visits Yes.*
- Select *Charges No.*
- Click *Go.*

2. In the *Date* column, locate the visit date for patient Darryl Smith's SNF charges from Activity 7-3. Then click on the *Charges* button on the right side of your screen for the date of service corresponding to Darryl's Activity 7-3 charges. (Remember, the *Charges* button may not necessarily appear in Darryl Smith's row; it may appear in the row of a different patient who has the same date of service.)

3. Then click *Go* on the left side of your screen. The charges for all patient encounters/ manual charges on the Date of Service (DOS) display. **Note:** You may receive a pop-up message that says "Transaction Date must be within Period Start and End Dates: (of the date of your batch)." Click *OK*, and the charges appear in the lower portion of your screen.

4. Scroll down to the bottom of the lower screen, and click *Save* on the bottom left. (**Note:** If more than one charge [e.g., multiple patient visits] appear on the date, the *Charges* will be saved for all patients.)

5. Important!! Wait until the "Transaction Saved" message appears before moving on. Then click *OK*. You will receive another pop-up stating "Bulk Charges Saved." Click *OK*.

6. With patient Darryl Smith in context, click on the *OI* ⬛ button on the *Name Bar.*

---

4. Click on *Payment* in the *Open Action* column for *Procedure* 99214 and the *Open Items* dialog box will display in the lower portion of the screen. Procedure 99214 is not a covered charge. A charge that is not covered will have the dollar amount of the not covered charge listed in the "Not Covered (DENIAL)" column of the EOB/RA.

5. Enter the "Not Covered (DENIAL)" information from Darryl Smith's EOB/RA (Source Document 7-3, found at the end of this activity) for Procedure 99214 as instructed below. Your completed screen should look like **Figure 7-48**.

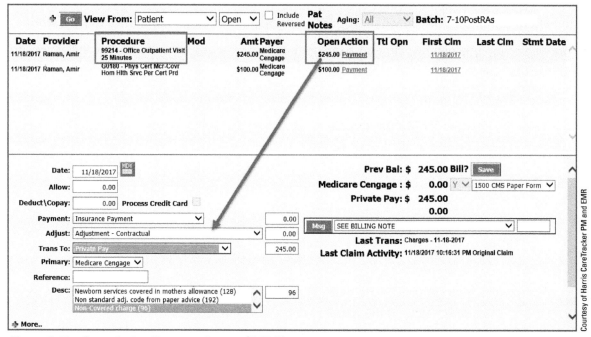

Figure 7-48   Open Action/Payment Screen $245 Charge

Note: Be sure to use the [Tab] key so that fields automatically populate.

    a. *Date*: Enter today's date (within the *Fiscal Period/Fiscal Year* set in your batch).

    b. *Allow*: Leave blank (0.00).

    c. *Deduct/Copay*: Leave blank (0.00).

    d. *Payment*: Using the drop-down, select "Insurance Payment." **Note:** You may need to change the field first to (Select Payment Type) and then back to "Insurance Payment." Be sure you use the [Tab] key so that amounts will populate in the proper fields.

    e. *Adjust*: Select (Select Adjustment); enter "0.00." Make sure this field is "0.00." If you need to enter "0.00," be sure you use the [Tab] key so that amounts will populate in the proper fields.

    f. *Transfer To*: Use the drop-down and select *Private Pay*. This will automatically populate the amount field to the right of *Trans To*, as well as the *Prev Bal* and *Private Pay* fields.

    g. *Primary*: Leave blank (or it can remain "Medicare Cengage").

    h. *Reference*: Leave blank.

    i. *Desc*: Type "96" in the blank box to the right of *Desc* and hit [Tab]. This will select "Non-Covered charge (96)."

    j. In the *Msg* field, use the drop-down list and select *SEE BILLING NOTE*.

    k. Your screen should reflect the same entries as noted in Source Document 7-3 for Procedure code 99214.

🖨 **Print the Not Covered (DENIAL) charge screen, label it "Activity 7-11a," and place it in your assignment folder.**

    l. Click *Save*. You will have to close out of the *OI* screen and re-open it before the claim disappears.

6. Click back on the *OI* button.

7. Enter the remittance information from Darryl Smith's EOB/RA (see Source Document 7-3 at the end of the activity) for Procedure G0180. Your completed screen should look like **Figure 7-49**.

8. In the *Open Items* window, click the *Payment* link under the *Action* header for the G0180 Procedure code charge. G0180 is a covered charge. **Note:** A covered charge will have <u>no</u> amount listed in the "Not Covered (DENIAL)" column of the EOB/RA. In the payment window on the lower part of the screen, enter the information from Darryl Smith's EOB/RA (Source Document 7-3).

    a. *Date:* Use today's date, the date you "received the EOB/RA" for the SNF charge you created in Activity 7-3.

    b. *Allow:* Enter the information from the *Amount Allowed* column on the EOB/RA (Source Document 7-3). Now hit the [Tab] button on your keyboard.

    c. *Deduct/Copay:* Enter the information from the *Deduct/Coins/Copay* column on the EOB/RA. Now hit the [Tab] button and this will populate the amount in the *Adjust* and *Transfer To* fields based on the information entered in the *Demographics* screen.

    d. *Payment*: Confirm that *Insurance Payment* is selected.

    e. *Adjust*: Confirm that *Adjustment—Contractual* is selected.

    f. *Trans To:* Confirm that *Private Pay* is selected.

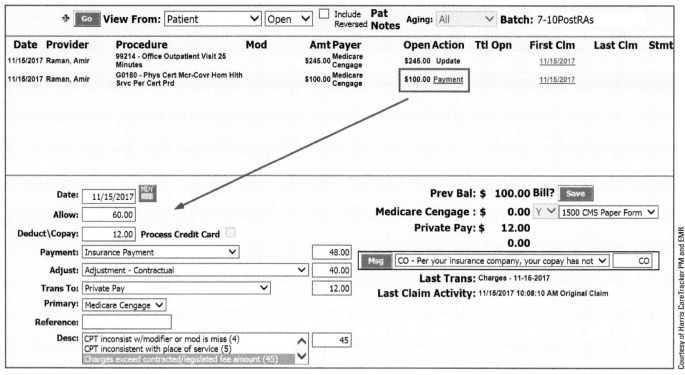

Figure 7-49   Open Action/Payment Screen $100 Charge

g. *Primary:* Confirm that *Medicare Cengage* is selected.

h. *Reference:* Leave blank.

i. *Desc:* Enter "45" in the blank box to the right of the *Desc* field, and hit the [Tab] key.

j. *Msg:* Enter "CO" in the blank box to the right of the drop-down menu and hit the *[Tab]* key.

🖨 **Print the Covered Charge screen, label it "Activity 7-11b," and place it in your assignment folder.**

9. Click *Save.*

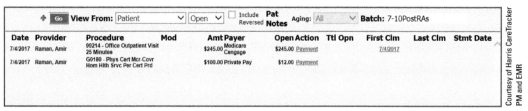

Figure 7-50   Denial and Remittance Information Saved—SNF Charge

10. You have now saved all the information from the EOB/RA related to the SNF charge you created in Activities 7-3 and 7-4 for Darryl Smith (as noted in **Figure 7-50**). You will have to close out of the *OI* screen and re-open it before the claim disappears.

11. Do **not** post the "7-10PostRAs" batch at this time. You will be instructed to post it later.

12. (FYI) Having entered the denial, the balance has now been transferred to private pay. **Note:** It is important to remember that it takes 24 hours for *Denials* to display in the *Dashboard* in a live environment. You can adjust your filters to set your display options. The *Dashboard* only shows *Denials* for the month.

Source Document 7-3   Explanation of Benefits/Remittance Advice

MEDICARE CENGAGE

Medicare Cengage
P.O. Box 234434
San Francisco, CA 94137

Date: MM/DD/YYYY (Date charge entered in Activity 7-3)
Payment Number: 5644712
Payment Amount: $ 48.00

AMIR RAMAN, D.O.
Napa Valley Family Health Associates (NVFHA)
101 Vine Street
Napa, CA 94558

Account Number	Patient Name				Subscriber Number			Claim Number			
Dates of Service	Description of Service	Amount Charged	Not Covered (DENIAL)	Prov Adj Discount	Amount Allowed	Deduct/ Coins/ Copay	Paid to Provider	Adj Reason Code	Rmk Code	Patient Resp
CARE1357	Smith, Darryl									
(Date charge entered in Activity 7-3)	G0180	$100.00		$ 40.00	$ 60.00	$12.00	$48.00	45*		$12.00
(Date charge entered in Activity 7-3)	99214	$245.00	$245.00			$245.00		96*		$ 245.00
TOTALS		$150.00	$245.00	$40.00	$60.00	$257.00	$48.00			$257.00

Amount Allowed (45*) = Charges exceed your contracted/legislated fee arrangement
Amount Allowed (20*) = Not a covered code

Current Procedural Terminology (C) 2018 American Medical Association

PROFESSIONALISM CONNECTION

For many patients and staff members, discussing the subject of money owed is touchy and uncomfortable. You must always address the topic in a calm and nonjudgmental way and comply with office policy, even if a patient requests special payment arrangements. Special requests should be documented and forwarded to the appropriate person or department, often the office manager, billing department, or managing provider. When asking for payment, use positive expressions. Practice your professionalism by role-playing with co-workers the following scenarios. Adjust the wording to your comfort level and to that of a service provider professional:

- When making an appointment by phone: "Copayment is expected at the time of service" or "Your office visit will be approximately $___. For your convenience we accept cash, checks, and credit card."

- For the patient checking in at the front desk: "Your copayment today will be $___."

- For patients checking out: "Your charges for today's office visit are $___. Would you like to pay by cash, check, or credit card?" or "I see your deductible has been met and/or insurance pays 80%. Your portion of the bill comes to $___. Would you like to pay by cash, check, or credit card?"

My challenge to you is to demonstrate how you would approach collection of payment in a positive and professional manner.

Activity 7-12
Work Credit Balances

Working credit balances by batch should be done immediately after an electronic remittance has been posted in Harris CareTracker PM. Credit balances are created when either a patient or an insurance company pays more money for a specific procedure for a specific date of service than what was billed. Credit balances can be identified by the *Credit Balances* link under the *Billing* section of the *Dashboard* in the *Home* module for a specific batch or group (**Figure 7-51**). After you post payments via electronic remittances, it is best practice to work credit balances for the batch you were working in before posting the batch.

There are two ways to work credit balances: *by Batch* or *for Refunds* (**Figure 7-52**). Once you post the batch, this will create a charge on the patient's account. You can then post a payment to create the credit balance.

TIP There is a big difference between a "Credit" and an "Unapplied Credit." A credit is an overpayment on an account, and an unapplied credit is only a patient payment (not insurance) that has not been attached to a DOS.

To Work Credit Balances:

In order to work a *Credit Balance*, you must first have a credit in the patient's account.

1. Pull patient Darryl Smith into context.

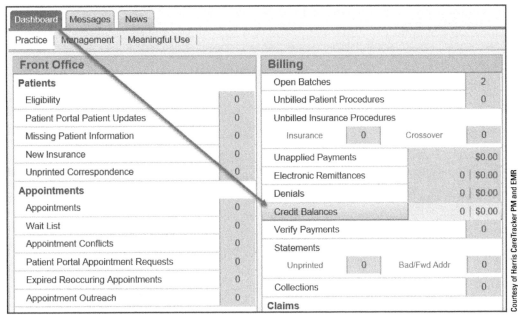

Figure 7-51   Credit Balances Link

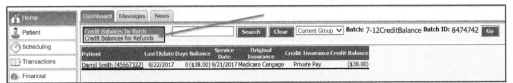

Figure 7-52   Work Credit Balances—by Batch or for Refunds   Courtesy of Harris CareTracker PM and EMR

2. Create a new batch and name it "7-12CreditBalance" using the following parameters:

   a. *Fiscal Period:* The fiscal period of Mr. Smith's SNF charge created in Activity 7-3.

   b. *Fiscal Year:* The fiscal year of Mr. Smith's SNF charge created in Activity 7-3.

   c. *Provider:* Select Mr. Smith's PCP (Dr. Raman).

   d. *Resource:* Select Dr. Raman as *Resource.*

   e. *Location:* Napa Valley Family Associates.

   f. Leave *Service Date From, Service Trans Date,* and *Payment Trans Date* blank.

3. Click *Save and Close* on the batch screen.

4. Click on the *OI* button on the *Name Bar.* Harris CareTracker PM displays the *Open Items* application.

5. To see a credit balance, you will need to post a payment to the patient's account first, following these instructions. The payment must be greater than the balance in the patient's account in *OI* in the *Open Action* column:

   a. Click on the *Payment* line in the *Open Action* column of his G0180 *Procedure* (which should be listed as "Private Pay" in the *Payer* column). The *payment* screen will display in the lower portion of the window.

   b. Using the *Payment* drop-down, select *Payment—Patient Cash (PATCSH).*

  c. In the amount field next to the *Payment* drop-down, enter a payment in the amount of $50.00. (**Note:** Do not enter the dollar sign.) You will see the *Private Pay* balance change to "$ –38.00" because the patient overpaid his copayment at checkin.

  d. Change the *Trans To* field to "Medicare Cengage."

  e. In the *Msg* drop-down select (or leave as) "Select Statement Message." Your screen should look like **Figure 7-53**.

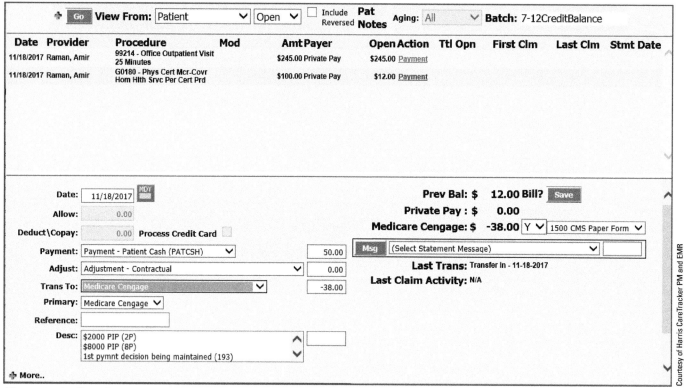

Figure 7-53   *Post Payment for Credit Balance*

  f. Click *Save*.

  g. To close the *Open Items* screen, click "X."

  h. Run a *Journal* for the "7-12CreditBalance" batch.

  i. *Post* the "7-12CreditBalance" batch.

6. Go to the *Home* module > *Dashboard* tab > *Billing* header > *Credit Balances* link (see Figure 7-51).

7. Click on the *Search* button and Harris CareTracker PM displays a list of open batches in the *Search* dialog box.

  a. Because you have already posted your batch, it does not display in the *Search* box.

  b. Type in "7-12" and click the "Includes Closed Batches" and "All Groups" checkboxes (**Figure 7-54**), and then click *Search*.

8. Click directly on the "7-12CreditBalance" batch line and it is pulled into context (**Figure 7-55**).

9. Click *Go* and Harris CareTracker PM displays a list of credit balances including the patient's name, the financial class with the credit balance, the amount of the credit, and the patient's last transaction date.

10. Pull patient Darryl Smith into context on the *Name Bar* if you have not already done so.

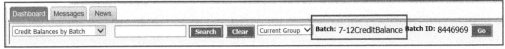

Figure 7-54   Include Closed Batches and All Groups to Work Credit Balances

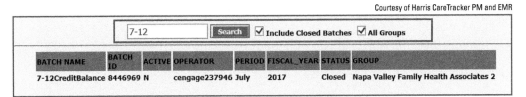

Figure 7-55   Pull 7-12 Batch into Context

11. In the drop-down menu found directly under the *Dashboard* tab, change "Credit Balances by Batch" to "Credit Balances for Refunds."

12. Since you posted the "7-12CreditBalance" batch previously in this activity, you will be prompted to create a new batch. Click *Edit* on the *Operator Encounter Batch Control.* Click *Create Batch.*

13. Create a batch using the following parameters:

    a. Name the new batch "7-12CrBalRefunds."

    b. Select the *Fiscal Period* and *Fiscal Year* of the SNF charge you created in Activity 7-3.

    c. Click *Save.*

    d. Confirm the entries in the batch control box (Provider/Resource/Location) and then click *Save and Close.*

    e. Your new batch has now been created.

14. Confirm that the date for the charge is included in the *Date From* and *Date To* fields. **Hint**: Always change the *Date To* field to include today's date.

15. Click *Go* and Mr. Smith's credit balance will pull in to the screen. (Refer to Step 14 **Hint** if the credit balance does not display.)

16. In the *Action* Column, use the drop-down and select *Refund-Patient (P)* (**Figure 7-56**).

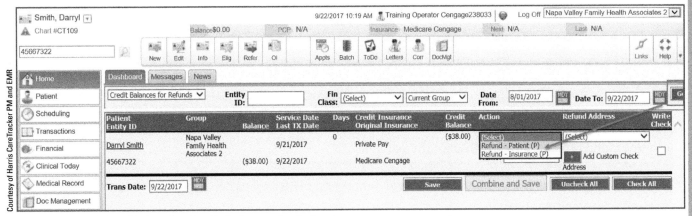

Figure 7-56   Select Patient for Credit Balances for Refunds

📠 **Print the Credit Balance for Refunds screen, label it "Activity 7-12," and place it in your assignment folder.**

17. Click *Save*.

18. The *Credit Balance Transfer* dialog box will display.

19. Click on *Write Transactions* (**Figure 7-57**).

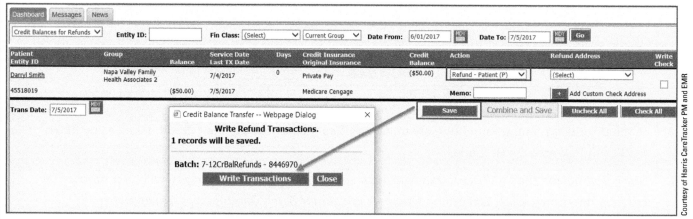

Figure 7-57   Write Transactions

20. The *Credit Balance Transfer* dialog box will confirm that the transaction has been saved (**Figure 7-58**).

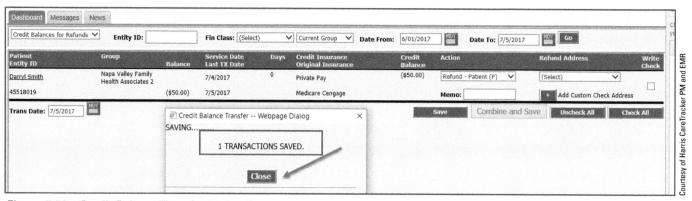

Figure 7-58   Credit Balance Transfer Dialog Box

21. Click *Close*, and the credit balance is removed from your screen.

Activity 7-13
Save Charges, Process Remittance, and Transfer to Private Pay

In order to continue with billing and collections activities, you must build and generate claims, save the charges, and process the EOB/RAs for the patient.

Before you begin, refer back to the patient encounter and record the date of the encounter for Alec Winfrey (Source Document 7-4): _____

1. Create a new batch and name it "7-13PostRAs" with the following parameters:

   a. Select the *Fiscal Period* and *Fiscal Year* for today's date.

   b. Click *Save*.

c. Leave the *Provider/Resource/Location* as is.

d. Click *Save and Close.*

TIP Since you have multiple batches open, it is best practice to confirm that you are working in the correct batch. To confirm, click on the *Batch* icon. The batch you are working in will display. If the batch displaying is NOT the batch you are instructed to be working in, click *Edit*, and in the *Operator Encounter batch control* box, use the drop down by each of the following batch fields (the *Encounter Batch Control*, *Payment Batch Control*, and *the Reversal Batch Control*), and change to the name of the batch you want to be working in. When finished click *Save and Close.* You will now be working in the different batch you selected.

---

2. Check that charges have been saved for patient Alec Winfrey. To do this, go to the *Home* module > *Dashboard* tab > *Visit* header > *Missing Encounters* > *Charges* link and set the fields as follows:

    • Change the beginning date to January 1, 20XX (current year) and change the ending date to today's date. Be sure the dates include the date of the patient's encounter.

    • Select *All providers*.

    • Select *All locations*.

    • Select *Visits Yes*.

    • Select *Charges No*.

    • Then click *Go.* You will see only *Charge(s)* that have <u>not</u> been saved. Charges for Alec Winfrey would have been saved in Activity 7-10 if his appointment was on the same date as Alison Wild (when you previously saved her charges). If the appointment was on a different date than Alison Wild's, then the charges for that appointment will appear here and the charges will need to be saved. If displaying, save the charges now. You can refer back to steps 8–12 of Activity 7-10 for assistance if needed. **Hint:** If no charges are displaying, move on to the next step.

3. Generate paper claims for all procedures listed for Mr. Winfrey (refer to the steps noted below):

    • Pull patient into context.

    • Click the *OI* tab in the *Name* bar.

    • Click on *Instant Claim* in the *First Clm* column (refer to Figure 7-31) for one of the procedures. Harris CareTracker PM displays the *Claims Summary* in the lower frame of the screen.

    • Place a check mark next to each claim and then click *Build Claim.* You will then note that the date you performed the activity is listed in the *First Clm* column.

4. Process the EOB/RA for Mr. Winfrey from Source Document 7-4 provided at the end of this activity. Refresher steps are provided as a "Tip."

TIP *Refresher:* Process an EOB/RA

1. If you are not already viewing the *Open Items* window, click on the *OI* button in the *Name Bar*.
2. Click on the *Payment* link in the *Action* column next to the Procedure(s).
3. Harris CareTracker PM displays the payment window in the lower frame of the screen (refer to **Figure 7-45**).

(continued)

4. In the payment window on the lower part of the screen, enter the information from the patient's EOB/RA (see the Source Documents provided at the end of this activity) for the *visit* as follows. First determine if the charge is covered or not covered. To do this, look in the "Not Covered (DENIAL)" column. A covered charge will have no amount listed in the "Not Covered (DENIAL)" column. A not covered charge has an amount listed in the "Not Covered (DENIAL)" column. As described below, the process you follow for entering the charge will vary depending on if the charge is covered or not covered. All charges for Alec are covered, therefore, follow the steps below:

Covered Charges

- *Date:* This should be today's date, the date you "received the EOB/RA" for the encounter for the patient visit.
- *Allow:* Enter the information from the *Amount Allowed* column on the EOB/RA. Now hit the [Tab] button on your keyboard.
- *Deduct/Copay:* Enter the information from the *Deduct/Coins/Copay* column on the EOB. Now hit the [Tab] button and this will populate the amount in the *Adjust* and *Transfer To* fields based on the information entered in the *Demographics* screen.
- *Payment:* Confirm that *Insurance Payment* is selected.
- *Adjust:* Confirm that *Adjustment—Contractual* is selected.
- *Trans To:* Confirm that *Private Pay* is selected.
- *Primary:* Confirm that the patient's correct insurance is selected.
- *Reference:* Leave blank.
- *Desc:* Leave as is.
- *Msg:* Leave as is.

5. Once you have entered the EOB/RA information, click *Save*. Your transaction will be saved and the claim disappears. (You have now saved all the entries from the EOB/RA related to the charge you created. You have to close out of the *OI* screen and re-open it before the claim disappears.)

6. If you were working multiple charges, you would repeat the steps to enter each of the charges listed on the EOB/RA. Refer to **Figure 7-46** for an example of what your screen looks like as you enter EOB/RAs.

7. Close out of the *Open Items* window by clicking the "X" in the upper-right corner of the window.

5. Upon completion of *ALL* payment/denial entries from the EOB/RA, run a *Journal* (reference Activity 7-5 for assistance) and review for accuracy. Do **not** post the "7-13PostRAs" batch at this time.

Print the Journal after completing all the 7-13 activities and label it "Activity 7-13 (a-c)," and place in your assignment folder.

Source Document 7-4 Explanation of Benefits

CENTURY MEDICAL PPO—CENGAGE

Century Medical PPO
PO Box 87542
San Jose, CA 95101

Date: MM/DD/YYYY (Appt. date used in Activity 4-1)
Payment Number: 212311
Payment Amount: $0.00

AMIR RAMAN, M.D.
Napa Valley Family Health Associates (NVFHA)
101 Vine Street
Napa, CA 94558

Current Procedural Terminology (C) 2018 American Medical Association

Account Number	Patient Name					Subscriber Number			Claim Number			
Dates of Service	Description of Service	Amount Charged	Not Covered (DENIAL)	Prov Adj Discount		Amount Allowed	Deduct/ Coins/ Copay	Paid to Provider	Adj Reason Code	Rmk Code	Patient Resp
CMED2478	Winfrey, Alec										
(Appt. date used in Activity 4-1)	99213	$112.00		$35.00		$77.00	$77.00	$0.00	45*		$42.00
(Appt. date used in Activity 4-1)	71020	$13.50		$3.50		$10.00	$10.00	$0.00	45*		$10.00
(Appt. date used in Activity 4-1)	36415	$15.00		$5.00		$10.00	$10.00	$0.00	45*		$10.00
(Appt. date used in Activity 4-1)	85025	$195.00		$95.00		$100.00	$100.00	$0.00	45*		$100.00
TOTALS		$335.50		$139.50		$197.00	$197.00	$0.00			$162.00

Amount Allowed (45*) = Charges exceed your contracted/legislated fee arrangement
Amount Allowed (22*) = (CO) Patient has not yet met annual policy deductible ($6,000.00). All balances are patient's responsibility.
Amount Allowed (25*) = Requires Modifier 25 to be paid as a separate service

CRITICAL THINKING There was a lot to cover in this chapter! Describe your understanding of the many different types of insurance plans and the effects on the practice when there is an issue regarding noncovered services.

    If you are tasked with communicating the fees for services to patients, collecting copays, or billing/collections on overdue accounts, describe what communication skills you would use. How would you incorporate empathy toward the patient while performing your financial responsibilities? How would using an electronic health record help with your duties? Write out some scenarios and practice on a family member, classmate, or friend.

PROFESSIONALISM CONNECTION

When Jim Mcginness checked in for his visit, the front desk clerk did not request a copy of his insurance card and did not verify his current information. Jim's employer had changed to a new Health Insurance plan since his last visit to NVFHA, and his claim will be rejected by his former insurance company because he was no longer covered by them. In addition, the amount of copay collected will be wrong.

a. How would you handle the situation?

b. How could it be avoided in the future?

c. Document all the steps required to be followed due to a failure to update information and copy the current insurance card.

d. Describe the impact on the revenue cycle to the practice.

e. Are there any other impacts?

f. Would the patient lose faith in NVFHA and wonder if issues affecting his health care would also be compromised?

Hint: As best practice, run an eligibility check before generating the claim to the insurance and update information as necessary.

CASE STUDIES

Case Study 7-1
Using patient Jim Mcginness:

1. Perform an *Eligibility Check* before generating a claim. Although *ClaimsManager* is not active in your student version of Harris CareTracker, for this simulated activity you note that Jim's claim will be denied. The original insurance recorded in his demographics returns an eligibility status of "ineligible" (current insurance no longer valid).

2. In this instance, you recall from Chapter 4 that Jim's insurance changed but was not updated at check-in. The normal workflow would be obtain updated insurance information and record it in his demographics. (**Note:** If the patient's visit had already been billed, it may require that it be rebilled to his visit to the new insurance company if necessary.)

3. Refer back to Chapter 4 and *Edit* Jim's demographics with new insurance information before proceeding to capture his visit with the following information:

   a. Deactivate Jim's former insurance company

   b. Add new insurance company: Blue Shield

   c. Subscriber #: BCBS987

   d. Eligible from: Use the first day of last month

   e. Copay: $20.00

Case Study 7-2

Build and generate a paper claim, save charges, and process the remittance for patient Harriet Oshea.

1. Create a new batch and name it "Ch7CS-Remit."

2. Repeat Activity 7-9 and build and generate paper claims for all procedures listed for Harriet.

3. Process the Proplan remittance (EOB/RA) (refer Activity 7-10) for her encounter using Source Document 7-5 (on the next page).

4. Upon completion, run a journal and review.

🖫 **Print the Journal, label it "Case Study 7-2," and place it in your assignment folder.**

5. Post the "Ch7CS-Remit" batch.

Source Document 7-5: Explanation of Benefits/Remittance Advice

PROPLAN

PROPLAN
P.O. Box 22315
Oakland, CA 94601

Date: xx/xx/20xx (use today's date)
Payment Number: 2344570
Payment Amount: $97.75

ANTHONY BROCKTON, M.D.
Napa Valley Family Health Associates (NVFHA)
101 Vine Street
Napa, CA 94558

Current Procedural Terminology (C) 2016 American Medical Association

Account Number	Patient Name				Subscriber Number			Claim Number			
Dates of Service	Description of Service	Amount Charged	Not Covered (DENIAL)	Prov Adj Discount	Amount Allowed	Deduct/ Coins/ Copay	Paid to Provider	Adj Reason Code	Rmk Code	Patient Resp	
9706416	OSHEA, HARRIET										
03/20/2017	99213	$112.00		$33.81	$78.19	$15.64**	$62.55	45*		$15.64	
03/20/2017	73520	$82.00		$56.00	$26.00	$5.20	$20.80	45*		$5.20	
03/20/2017	73565	$63.00		$45.00	$18.00	$3.60	$14.40	45*		$3.60	
03/20/2017	36415	$15.00	$15.00		$0.00	$15.00	$0.00	96*		$15.00	

Amount Allowed (45*) = Charges exceed your contracted/legislated fee arrangement
Amount Allowed (20*) = Not a covered code
Amount Allowed (25*) = requires Modifier 25 to be paid as a separate service

ClaimsManager and Collections

Learning Objectives

1. Use the features of ClaimsManager in Harris CareTracker PM and EMR.
2. Check status and work unpaid/inactive claims.
3. Generate patient statements.
4. Review collection status and transfer private pay balances.
5. Create collection letters.
6. Generate collection letters.

Real-World Connection

It cannot be overstated that all personnel, including office staff or collections agents, must act with the utmost professionalism during the collection process. Not only do numerous laws and regulations apply to the collection process, but also the sensitive nature of the relationship between provider and patient must be protected. Credit information of the patient is considered confidential and may not be released without the patient's expressed permission. Financial information regarding the patient is also confidential and must be protected according to the law. Both in-person and telephone discussions should be conducted in an area that is out of view and hearing of other patients.

Credit arrangements and interest charges must be disclosed in writing. Enforcing the credit policy can be uncomfortable for both patients and staff. You must overcome any inhibitions regarding discussion of fees and payments. The success of the practice relies heavily on the medical assistant's ability to politely yet firmly ask for payment from patients. The first step in the collection process is to advise patients of the office policy regarding payment when they call to schedule an appointment. It is important that you remain calm, compassionate, and empathetic to patients. If you encounter a difficult patient, follow these steps to diffuse and resolve the matter:

1. Let the patient vent.
2. Express empathy to the patient. The tone of your voice goes a long way. Use a genuinely warm and caring tone to enhance the meaning of empathetic phrases.
3. Begin problem-solving. Ask the patient questions to help clarify the situation and cause of the problem and double-check the facts.
4. Mutually agree on the solution. Be careful not to make a promise you cannot keep.
5. Follow up. You will score big points by following up with your patient to resolve the problem. This is sometimes referred to as service recovery.

You must demonstrate professionalism with every contact and treat each patient with the utmost respect. Your collection activities should be client-oriented and demonstrate the proper attitude and temperament with close attention given to protecting the goodwill established with your patient. Let me challenge you to role-play with your co-workers various collection scenarios that you might encounter. This will help with preparedness, conveying empathy, and noting the tone and inflection in your voice.

Before you begin the activities in this chapter, refresh your memory on working with Harris CareTracker by referring back to the Best Practices list on page xiv of this workbook. This list is also posted to the student companion website. Following best practices will help you complete work quickly and accurately.

CLAIMSMANAGER

Learning Objective 1: Use the features of Claims Manager in Harris CareTracker PM and EMR.

The *ClaimsManager* application in Harris CareTracker PM electronically screens a claim and the associated CPT®, ICD, and HCPCS codes and modifiers at the time the claim is created.

Activity 8-1
Work the Claims Worklist

Most claims are sent electronically in Harris CareTracker PM. Any claims identified with a problem that would prevent them from being paid will show up on a *Claims Worklist* to be resolved. The *Claims Worklist* identifies the following:

- Newly prepared claims that will be transmitted during your next claim run
- Claims that cannot be transmitted electronically due to a missing submitter number
- Claims that cannot be transmitted from Harris CareTracker PM because of missing information
- Claims that are not transmitted because of errors identified by *ClaimsManager*
- Claims that will not be accepted by a payer because of missing information
- Claims that you manually flagged as missing information or in review
- Claims that a payer does not have on file and claims with a denial status

Any claims flagged in any of the *Claims Worklist* columns, except *New/Prepared*, need to be followed up on, which typically requires you to add and/or edit information and rebill the claim. Harris CareTracker PM performs an electronic claim status check and, based on its status, moves the claim to one of the *Claims Worklist* categories. You can also manually flag a claim to move it to a *Claims Worklist* category.

The *Claims Worklist* is grouped into four main categories: *New/Prepared*, *Claim Errors*, *Pending*, and *Other* (**Figure 8-1**).

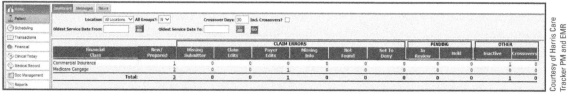

Figure 8-1   Claims Worklist Categories

The *Claim Summary* screen (**Figure 8-2**) displays when an individual claim line is clicked. In this screen, actions can be performed on the selected claim only.

To Work the Claims Worklist:

1. Go to the *Home* module > *Dashboard* tab > *Billing* section > *Claims Worklist* link. There are three options: *Unbilled*, *Crossover*, and *Inactive* (**Figure 8-3**). Select *Unbilled*. This will take you to the *Claims Worklist* screen.

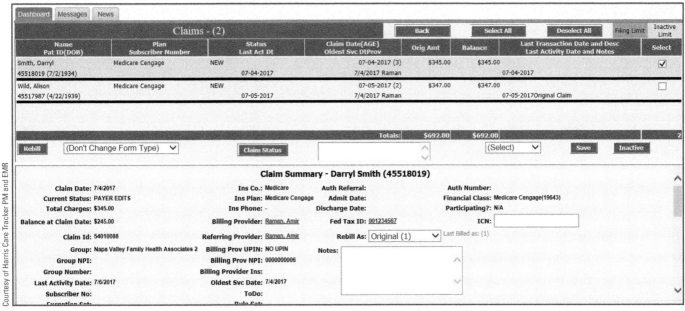

Figure 8-2   Claims Summary Screen

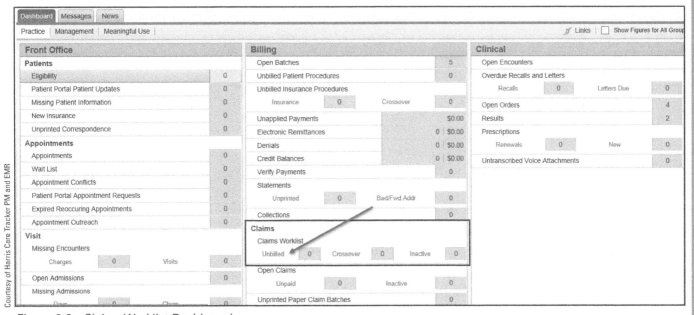

Figure 8-3   Claims Worklist Dashboard

2. The *Location* list defaults to "All Locations." You have the option to select a specific location if needed. Leave as is.

3. The *All Groups* list defaults to "N" for No. Select "Y" for Yes if you want to include claims for all groups. Select "Y."

4. Enter "180" in the *Crossover Days* field.

5. Select the *Incl. Crossovers?* checkbox to include crossover claims.

6. Leave the *Oldest Service Date From/To* as is. If you wanted to view claims from a specific time period, you would enter a date range here.

7. Click *Go.* The application displays a list of all claims broken down by financial class (**Figure 8-4**).

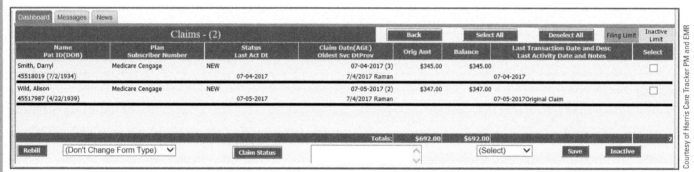

Figure 8-4   Claims by Financial Class

8. Click on a number in the *New/Prepared* column for the corresponding financial class you need to work (select the column for "Medicare Cengage"). The *New/Prepared Claims* screen will display (**Figure 8-5**).

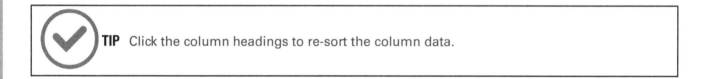

Figure 8-5   New/Prepared Claims Screen

✓ **TIP** Click the column headings to re-sort the column data.

---

9. Select the checkbox in the *Select* column for each claim you want to work. Select the first claim for Darryl Smith by clicking directly in his claim summary line (the claim summary line is the line that contains the patient's name and claim information). The claim line now appears in yellow and the application displays the *Claim Summary* in the lower frame of the screen (see Figure 8-2).

10. Scroll down on the lower portion of the screen and then click the *Claim Status* button. You will receive a pop-up (**Figure 8-6**) advising you of the claim's status (which displays "Processing. . . ."). **Do NOT** click the *Close* button in the pop-up as this will remove the claim from the *Unbilled Claims* screen. Rather, click on the "X" in the upper-right-hand corner to close out of the window.

11. Now click directly in the claim summary line containing Darryl Smith's first visit again to display the *Claim Summary* in the lower frame of the screen (see Figure 8-2). This allows you to review, edit, check claim status, or rebill an individual claim.

12. Scroll down and look under the *Activity Notes* column to determine the inaccurate or missing claim information that, triggered by *ClaimsManager*, prevented the claim from being transmitted from Harris CareTracker PM, that prevented the claim from being accepted by a payer, or that caused the claim to be denied by the payer (**Figure 8-7**).

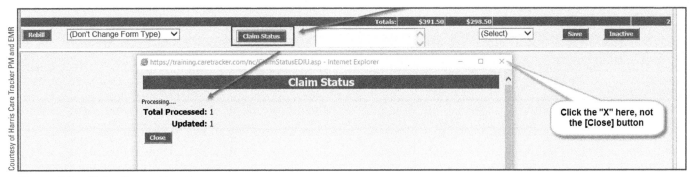

Figure 8-6   Claim Status Pop-Up

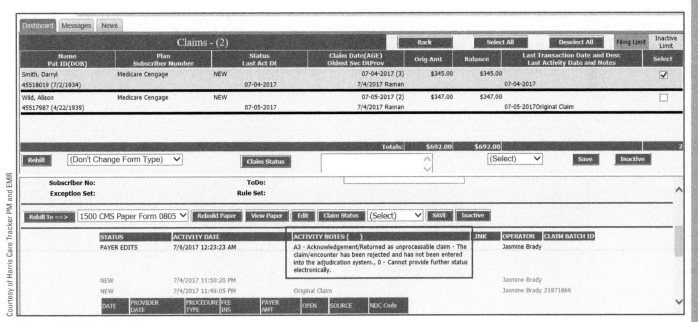

Figure 8-7   Activity Notes

13. Perform the desired action on the claim(s):

Confirm that *Billing Provider* and *Referring Provider* displays Dr. Raman. If not, scroll down and click *Edit* on the *Claim Summary* screen (**Figure 8-8**). The *Claim Transaction Summary* window displays the location, place of service, encounter-specific claim information, referring provider, diagnosis code, and modifiers. Click *Save* (**Figure 8-9**). You may briefly receive an "error" message. Click *OK*. Your *Claim Summary* will now reflect the update to *Referring Provider*.

TIP

• When the billing provider, dates of service, procedure codes, fee, units, servicing provider, or insurance need to be changed, the charge must be reversed from Harris CareTracker PM via the *Edit* application in the *Transactions* module. The charge will then be put back into the system.

• When rebilling claims, the form type is not typically changed.

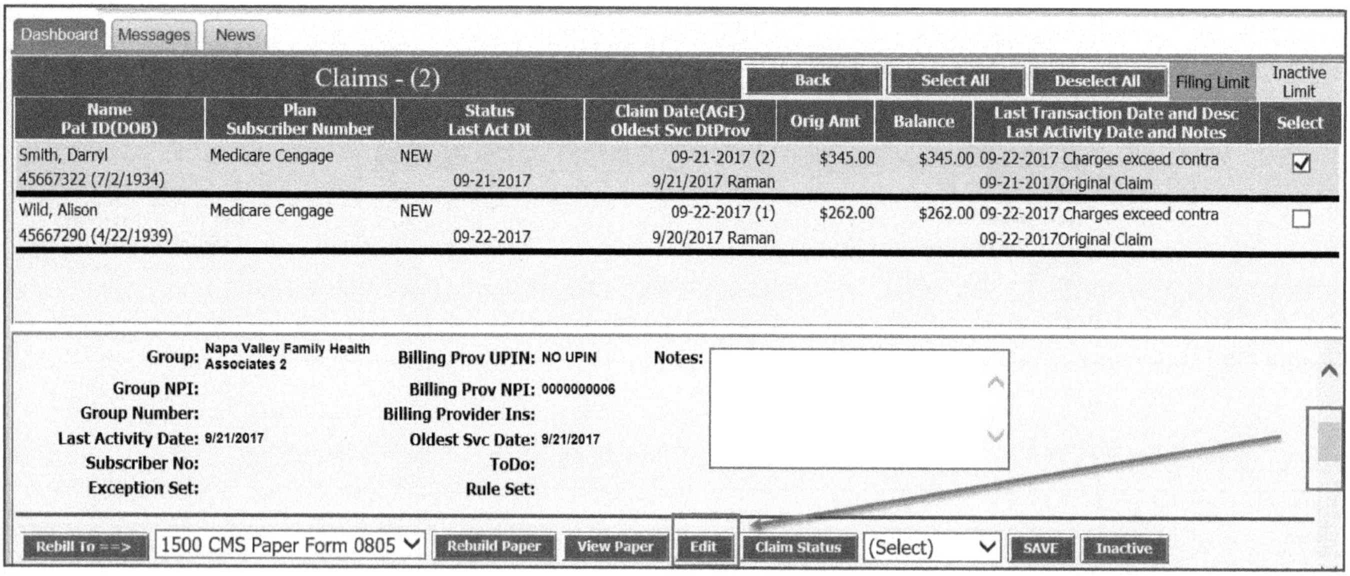

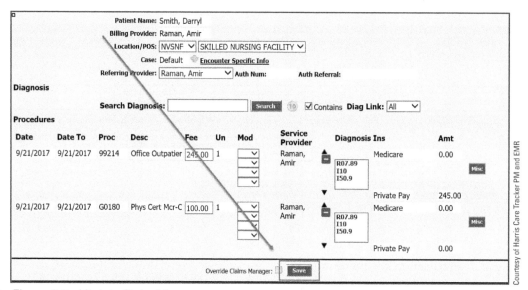

Figure 8-8   Edit Claim Summary

Figure 8-9   Update Claim Message

14. Now select the same claim by clicking in the claim summary line again (which will turn yellow) and checking the *Select* box even if there were no edits (the only "edit" noted in step 12 was to confirm or change the *Billing Provider* and *Referring Provider* to Dr. Amir Raman).

15. Now, scroll down and click *Rebill To ==>*. Harris CareTracker PM places the claim in the *New/Pending* category of the *Claims Worklist* and the claim will be transmitted during the next claim run.

16. Scroll down the screen and in the *Activity Notes* column, you will now see the activities completed (**Figure 8-10**).

📇 **Print the Claim Status Activity screen, label it "Activity 8-1," and place it in your assignment folder.**

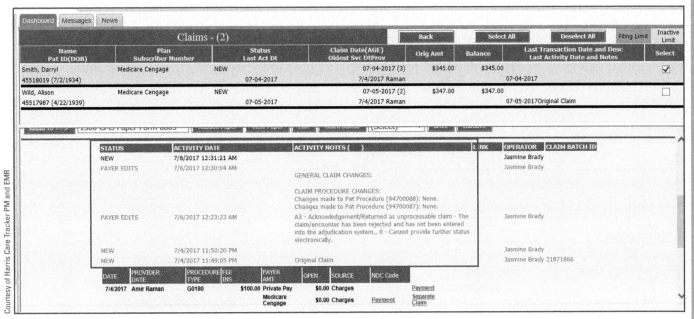

Figure 8-10   Claims Status Activity Note

Activity 8-2

Search Crossover Claims

A crossover claim is a claim that is automatically forwarded from Medicare to a secondary insurer after Medicare has paid its portion of a service.

1. Go to the *Home* module > *Dashboard* tab > *Billing* section > *Claims Worklist* link. Select *Crossover* from the three options. Harris CareTracker PM opens the *Claims Worklist* application.

2. The *Location* list defaults to "All Locations." Leave as is.

3. The *All Groups* list defaults to "N" for No. Select "Y" for Yes to include claims for all groups.

4. Adjust the crossover days to 180.

5. Select the *Incl. Crossovers?* checkbox.

6. Leave the *Oldest Service Date From/To* as is. If you wanted to view claims from a specific time period, you would enter a date range here.

7. Click *Go*. Harris CareTracker PM displays a list of all claims organized by financial class (**Figure 8-11**).

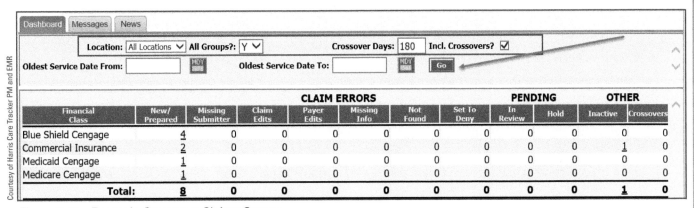

Figure 8-11   Example Crossover Claims Screen

💾 **Print the Crossovers search screen, label it "Activity 8-2," and place it in your assignment folder.**

8. If there are crossover claims noted in the *Crossovers* column, click the number that corresponds to the financial class in which you want to work. Harris CareTracker PM displays a list of crossover claims (**Figure 8-12**). Hint: There are no *Crossover Claims* for you to work here.

Courtesy of Harris Care Tracker PM and EMR

Dashboard	Messages	News

Location: [All Locations ▾] All Groups?: [N ▾]   Crossover Days: [180] Incl. Crossovers? ☑
Oldest Service Date From: [____] 📅   Oldest Service Date To: [____] 📅   [Go]

Financial Class	New/ Prepared	Missing Submitter	Claim Edits	Payer Edits	Missing Info	Not Found	Set To Deny	In Review	Hold	Inactive	Crossovers
				CLAIM ERRORS				PENDING		OTHER	
Commercial Insurance	3	0	0	0	0	0	0	0	0	1	0
Medicare Cengage	2	0	0	0	0	0	0	0	0	0	0
Total:	**5**	**0**	**0**	**0**	**0**	**0**	**0**	**0**	**0**	**1**	**0**

Figure 8-12   *Crossover Claims Displayed*

💡 **FYI** In a live environment, you would do the following:

a. In the *Bill?* column, select the checkbox next to each claim you want to bill to secondary insurance. Alternatively, click *Check All* to bill all claims as crossover claims.

b. Click *Set to Bill*. All crossover claims are saved as Secondary 1500 Forms under the *Unprinted Paper Claims* link for printing in the next bill run.

WORK UNPAID CLAIMS

Learning Objective 2: Check status and work unpaid/inactive claims.

Activity 8-3
Individually Check Claim Status Electronically

Harris CareTracker PM automatically checks the status of unpaid claims every evening with specific payers and will check the status of all claims with an outstanding balance. When a check is complete, the claim's status is updated, attached to the claims, and if necessary will also be flagged in *Claims Worklist* if a status of "Not Found," "Set to Deny," or "In Review" is returned.

Claim status is automatically checked every evening for every claim that has an outstanding balance. Typically, a manual claim status check is not necessary. However, if you need to manually check claim status, you do so individually or in a batch.

Claim status for individual claims can be checked from any application in Harris CareTracker PM where the *Claim Summary* screen displays.

1. Go to the *Home* module > *Dashboard* tab > *Billing* section > *Open Claims/Unpaid* link. Harris CareTracker PM displays the *Open Claims* application.

2. Select the desired filter options, as outlined (**Figure 8-13**):

   a. *Status*: NEW

   b. *Age By*: Oldest Service Date

   c. *Financial Class*: Leave as is

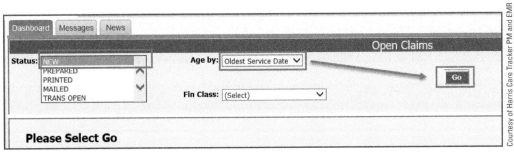

Figure 8-13   Unpaid Claims Link

3. Click *Go*. Harris CareTracker PM displays the *Unpaid/Inactive* claims, broken down by financial class and by week. The total inactive claims for a financial class displays in the *Inactive* column. Totals for all unpaid claims for a financial class displays in the *Total* column, and for each week, the total number of unpaid claims displays in the *Totals* row (**Figure 8-14**).

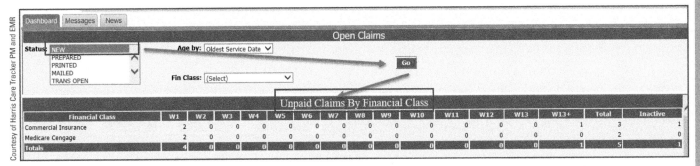

Figure 8-14   Open Claims

4. To work the "Commercial Insurance" *Financial Class* claims, click on the corresponding number in the *Total* column of *Commercial Insurance*. Harris CareTracker PM displays a claim line for all corresponding *Unpaid/Inactive* claims with the patient's name, ID number, date of birth, subscriber number, the insurance plan for which the claim was transmitted, the claim status, last activity date on the claim, claim date, claim age, oldest service date on the claim, the provider on the claim, the original amount, balance remaining, and the last activity notes saved for the claim.

5. Place a check mark in Alec Winfrey's *Select* column.

6. Then click directly on the patient's claim line. The line turns yellow and Harris CareTracker PM displays the *Claim Summary* in the lower frame of the screen.

7. You may need to scroll down the screen to be able to view the claim summary (**Figure 8-15**). Click *Claim Status*.

8. When the *Claim Status* window has finished processing, close out of it by clicking only the "X" in the upper-right corner (do **not** click on the *Close* button).

9. Re-select the claim by directly clicking on the patient's claim line.

10. You must scroll down and click the *Claim Status* button just above *Activity Notes* (**Figure 8-16**).

11. Click on the *Claims Status* button in the *Claim Status History* pop-up box. Harris CareTracker PM displays the *Claim Status History* window (**Figure 8-17**), which includes all previous status checks that have occurred, including the date of the status check, the operator who performed the check, the claim status category, and the *Claim Status* code. (**Note**: If the message says no history, close the box and click it again.)

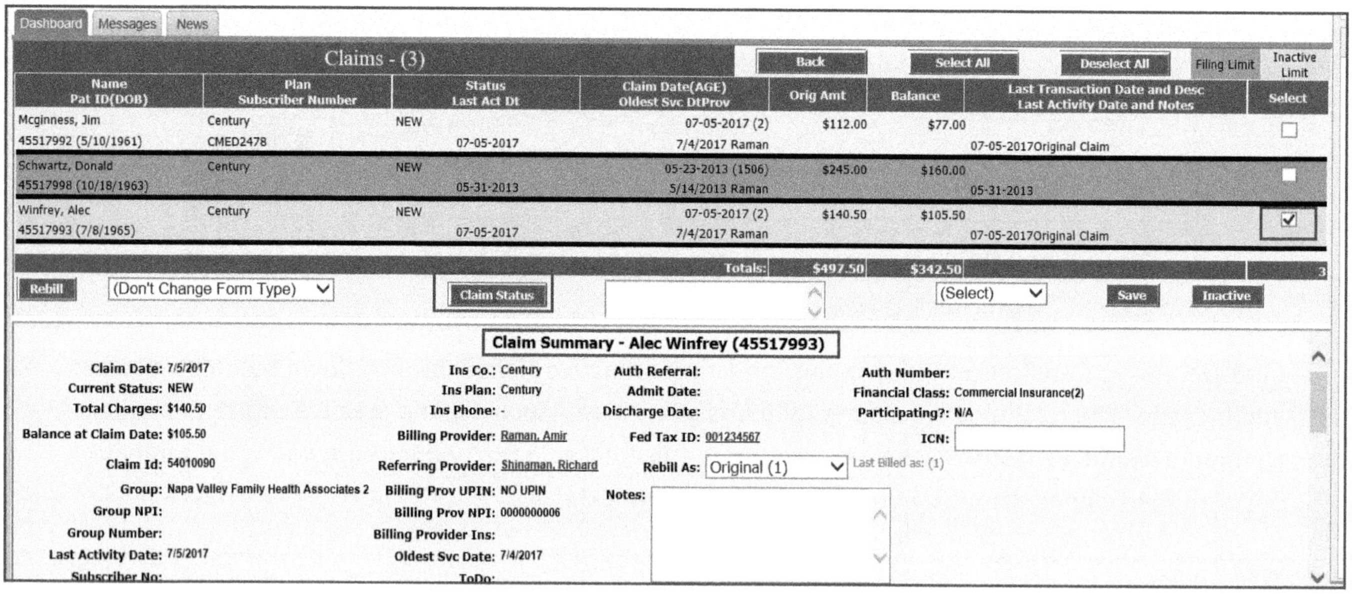

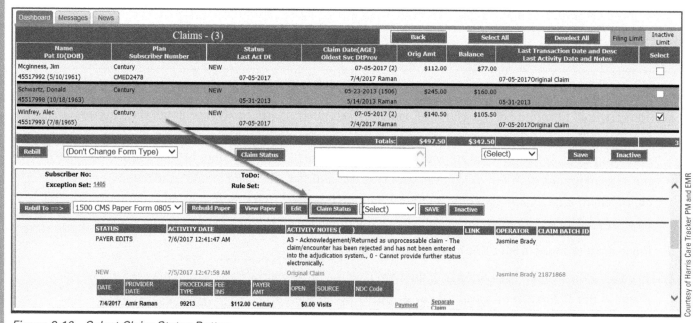

Figure 8-15   Claim Summary

Figure 8-16   Select Claim Status Button

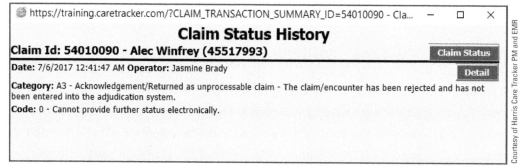

Figure 8-17   Claim Status History

12. Click on the *Claim Status* button on the top right corner of the *Claim Status History* window to perform another claim status check. When the claim status check is complete, the status of the current claim is automatically updated. Close out of the *Claim Status* box by clicking on the *Close* button.

13. To view the details of the check, click on the *Detail* button in the *Claim Status History* box, and the *Claim Status Detail* dialog box displays (**Figure 8-18**). (**Note:** The *Claim Status Detail* displayed will not match your patient, provider, and insurance. That is because this is an educational environment.)

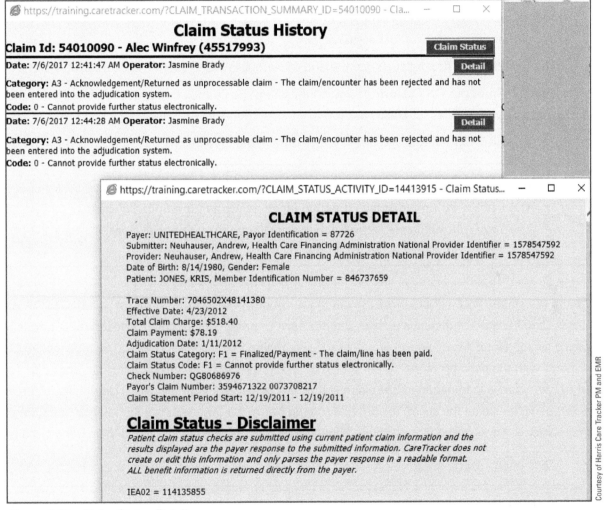

Figure 8-18   Claim Status Detail

 TIP When a claim's status has been returned, except for "Set to Pay," the claim will be moved to the corresponding column on the *Claims Worklist* screen.

📠 **Print the Claim Status Detail screen, label it "Activity 8-3," and place it in your assignment folder.**

14. Click "X" in the top right corner of the *Claim Status Detail* and the *Claim Status History* windows to close out of them.

Activity 8-4
Work Unpaid/Inactive Claims

Now that you have checked the claim status, begin working the unpaid/inactive claims. The steps are similar to checking a claim status, but you are now working the claim.

1. Go to the *Home* module > *Dashboard* tab > *Billing* section > *Open Claims/Unpaid* link.

2. Harris CareTracker PM displays the *Open Claims* application. Enter the following:

    a. *Status* field: Do not make a selection; leave as is. (**FYI**) The *Status* field is where you select the status of the claims you want to view. To select multiple statuses, you would press the *[Ctrl]* key while clicking to select multiple statuses.

    b. In the *Age by* drop-down list, select the age of claims to view. Select "Oldest Service Date."

    c. (Optional) From the *Fin Class* drop-down list, select the financial class containing the claims you want to view. Leave as "(Select)."

    d. Click *Go.* Harris CareTracker PM displays the unpaid/inactive claims by financial class and by week.

> **TIP** Unpaid claims by financial class:
> - The *Inactive* column displays the total inactive claims for a financial class.
> - The *Total* column displays the total unpaid claims for a financial class.
> - The *Totals* row displays the total unpaid claims for each week.

3. Locate the claims you want to work. Select the number in the *Total* column for "Medicare Cengage." Harris CareTracker PM displays a claim line for each unpaid/inactive claim. (**Note:** You cannot click on a zero total.) (**Note:** When a number is clicked, a claim line for all corresponding *Unpaid/Inactive Claims* displays with the patient's name, ID number, date of birth, subscriber number, the insurance plan for which the claim was transmitted, the claim status, last activity date on the claim, claim date, claim age, oldest service date on the claim, the provider on the claim, the original amount, balance remaining, and the last activity notes saved for the claim (**Figure 8-19**). Claims that have reached their *Filing Limit* will display in red.)

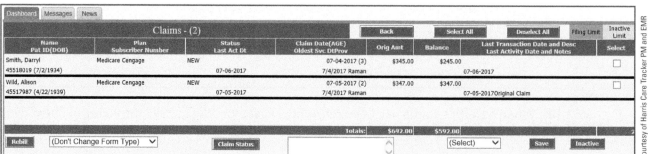

Figure 8-19   Unpaid/Inactive Claims

> **TIP** To work claims in a batch:
> - To work all claims, click *Select All* to select all of the claims.

4. To review or work an individual claim, click directly on the claim summary line (select Alison Wild's first claim). The claim line will turn yellow. Harris CareTracker PM displays the *Claim Summary* in the lower frame of the screen.

5. You will need to scroll down on both the upper and lower screens to view all the claims and the *Claim Summary* information for the claim selected.

6. Scroll down and click *Edit* on the *Claim Summary* screen (**Figure 8-20**) to change the location, place of service, encounter-specific claim information, referring provider, diagnosis code, and modifiers. The *Claim Transaction Summary* window displays (**Figure 8-21**), where you can make changes. **Note:** Dates of service, procedure codes, fees, the insurance company, and the amount of the claim may not be edited from this window.

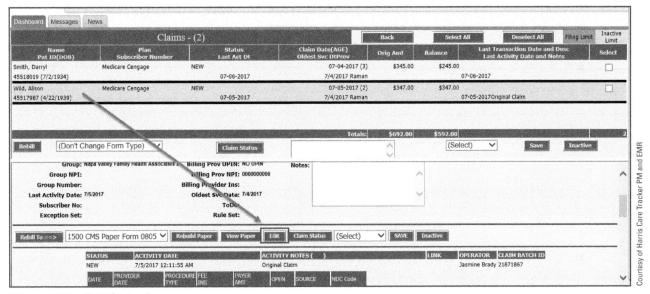

Figure 8-20   Edit Claim Summary

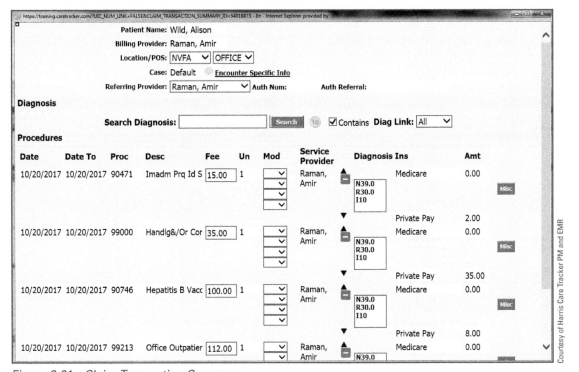

Figure 8-21   Claim Transaction Summary

7. Click on the [+] icon next to *Encounter Specific Info* and a pop-up *Preferred Patient Case* dialog box will appear. In the *Claim Information* tab, use the drop-down arrow and select "Dr. Raman" as both the *Supervising* and *Ordering Provider* (**Figure 8-22**).

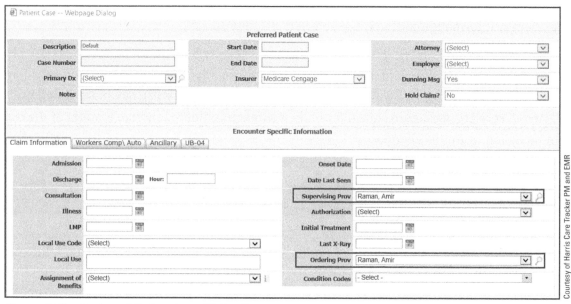

Figure 8-22   Preferred Patient Case Dialog Box

8. If you see a *Save For Charge* button, click on it, and the dialog box disappears and the screen returns to the *Encounters* dialog box. If no *Save For Charge* button is displaying, click "X" to close out of the dialog box.

9. Then click the *Save* button at the bottom of the *Claim Transaction Summary* dialog box and it will close. **Hint:** If the box does not "close" automatically, click on the "X" to close the dialog box.

TIP If there is a number in *Rule Set,* click the number link next to *ACTIVITY NOTES* to view descriptions of the rules for the insurance company. This can be helpful when determining the information that needs to be fixed. Click the *Key* link (in blue) (**Figure 8-23**) next to the *Activity Notes* heading to view a key for deciphering each missing information code (shown in **Figure 8-24**).

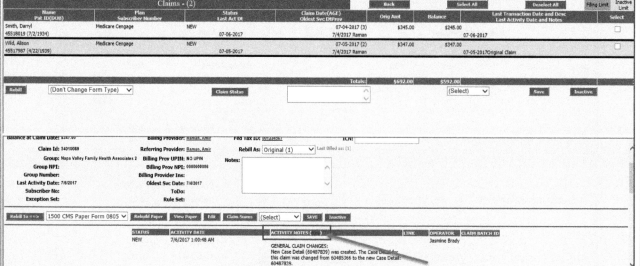

Figure 8-23   Rule Set

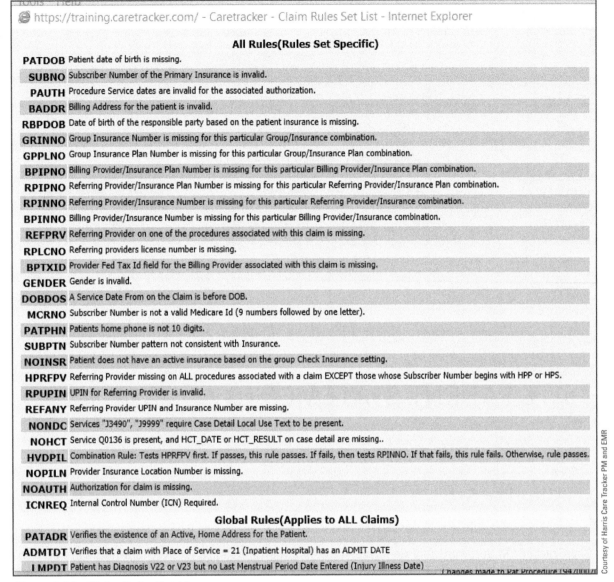

Figure 8-24   Claim Rules Set List

10. Scroll down the *Claim Summary* and click *Rebill To ==>*. Harris CareTracker PM will place the claim in the *New/Pending* category of the *Claims Worklist* screen and will transmit the claim during the next bill run (**Figure 8-25**). When rebilling claims, the form type typically is not changed.

Dashboard	Messages	News							

Claims - (2)				Back	Select All	Deselect All	Filing Limit	Inactive Limit

Name Pat ID(DOB)	Plan Subscriber Number	Status Last Act Dt	Claim Date(AGE) Oldest Svc DtProv	Orig Amt	Balance	Last Transaction Date and Desc Last Activity Date and Notes	Select
Smith, Darryl 45518019 (7/2/1934)	Medicare Cengage	NEW 07-06-2017	07-04-2017 (3) 7/4/2017 Raman	$345.00	$245.00	07-06-2017	☐
Wild, Alison 45517987 (4/22/1939)	Medicare Cengage	NEW 07-05-2017	07-05-2017 (2) 7/4/2017 Raman	$347.00	$347.00	07-05-2017Original Claim	☐

Claim Summary - Alison Wild (45517987)

Claim Date: 7/5/2017

Current Status: NEW

Total Charges: $347.00

Balance at Claim Date: $0.00

Claim Id: 54010089

Group: Napa Valley Family Health Associates 2

Ins Co.: Medicare

Ins Plan: Medicare Cengage

Ins Phone: -

Billing Provider: Raman, Amir

Referring Provider: Raman, Amir

Billing Prov UPIN: NO UPIN

Auth Referral:

Admit Date:

Discharge Date:

Fed Tax ID: 001234567

Rebill As: Original (1)   Last Billed as: (1)

Notes:

Auth Number:

Financial Class: Medicare Cengage(19643)

Participating?: N/A

ICN:

Courtesy of Harris Care Tracker PM and EMR

Figure 8-25   Last Transaction Update

 Print the Unpaid/Inactive screen, label it "Activity 8-4," and place it in your assignment folder.

GENERATE PATIENT STATEMENTS

Learning Objective 3: Generate patient statements.

Activity 8-5

Generate Patient Statements

Harris CareTracker PM automatically generates patient statements each week. Statements are sent to responsible parties who owe a private pay balance.

A statement will not be generated for a patient if the patient has an unapplied balance saved on his or her account that is equal to or greater than the patient's current balance amount.

Patient statements will not be generated by Harris CareTracker PM until 5 p.m., regardless of when you submit the request (**Figure 8-26**)

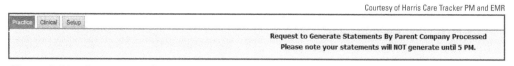

Courtesy of Harris Care Tracker PM and EMR

Practice	Clinical	Setup

Request to Generate Statements By Parent Company Processed
Please note your statements will NOT generate until 5 PM.

Figure 8-26   Statements Generate at 5 p.m.

1. Before beginning this activity, post the following batches: "7-12CrBalRefunds," "7-10PostRAs," and "SmithSNF."

2. With patient Alison Wild in context, go to the *Administration* module > *Practice* tab > *Daily Administration* section > *Financial* header > *Generate Statements* link (**Figure 8-27**). If a patient is in context, the application displays the option to generate statements for the parent company or the responsible party. You can generate statements for only the parent company when no patient is in context.

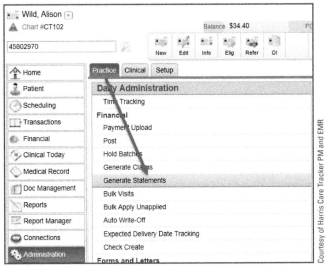

Figure 8-27   Generate Statements Link

3. In the *Generate Statements for Responsible Party* field, select the responsible party for whom you want to generate statements (select patient Alison Wild) and then click *Go!* (**Figure 8-28**).

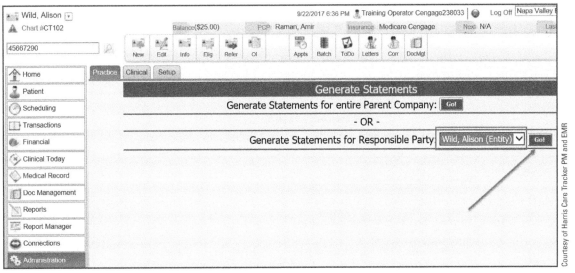

Figure 8-28   Generate Statements for Responsible Party—Alison Wild

4. The application schedules the statements to be printed. Your screen will look like **Figure 8-29**.

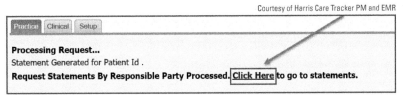

Figure 8-29   Statement Generated

SPOTLIGHT   If no statements are displaying, recheck after 24 hours (or after 5 p.m. on the date the activity is performed). Continue with your activities, and repeat Activity 8-5 in 24 hours.

5. Click on the blue "Click Here" prompt (see Figure 8-29) to go to the statements. **Note**: You may need to click on *Generate* and *Click Here* (in blue) again for the statement(s) to appear. If you receive an error message, click out of the *Administration* module and repeat the activity steps. Your screen will now look like **Figure 8-30**. (**Note**: If no results are showing, change the *Date Range* to "All Dates.")

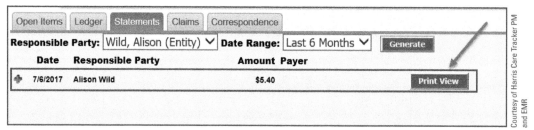

Figure 8-30   Statements Display

6. Click on the *Print View* button. The patient's statement will display in a new window (**Figure 8-31**).

7. Print the statement by right-clicking on the screen and selecting *Print* from the drop-down menu or by clicking the Print icon in the upper-right-hand corner.

🖶 Print

Napa Valley Family Associates

RESP PARTY ACCT #	109909-45802970	STMT DATE	11/19/2017
LAST PMT	$0	STMT TOTAL	$34.40

Statement - Page 1

DATE OF SERVICE	PATIENT	DESCRIPTION OF SERVICES	PROCEDURE CODE	SERVICING PROVIDER	AMOUNT	PATIENT AMT DUE
11/17/2017	Wild, Alison (45802970)	Office Outpatient Visit 15 Minutes	99213	Raman, Amir	$112.00	$14.40
		Per Your Insurance Company, Your Copay Has Not Been Paid In Full. The Balance Is Your Responsibility. Thank You.				
		Transaction 11/18/2017, Insurance Payment			-$57.60	
		Transaction 11/18/2017, Adjustment - Contractual			-$40.00	
		Transaction 11/18/2017, Charges exceed contracted/legislated fee amount				
11/17/2017	Wild, Alison (45802970)	Hepatitis B Vaccine Adult Dosage Intramuscular	90746	Raman, Amir	$100.00	$8.00
		Per Your Insurance Company, Your Copay Has Not Been Paid In Full. The Balance Is Your Responsibility. Thank You.				
		Transaction 11/18/2017, Insurance Payment			-$32.00	
		Transaction 11/18/2017, Adjustment - Contractual			-$60.00	
		Transaction 11/18/2017, Charges exceed contracted/legislated fee amount				
11/17/2017	Wild, Alison (45802970)	Handlg&/Or Convey Of Spec For Tr Office To Lab	99000	Raman, Amir	$35.00	$35.00
		See Billing Note				
		Transaction 11/18/2017, Non-Covered charge				
11/17/2017	Wild, Alison (45802970)	Imadm Prq Id Subq/Im Njxs 1 Vaccine	90471	Raman, Amir	$15.00	$2.00
		Per Your Insurance Company, Your Copay Has Not Been Paid In Full. The Balance Is Your Responsibility. Thank You.				
		Transaction 11/18/2017, Insurance Payment			-$8.00	
		Transaction 11/18/2017, Adjustment - Contractual			-$5.00	
		Transaction 11/18/2017, Charges exceed contracted/legislated fee amount				

Figure 8-31   Patient Statement

📋 **Print the patient statement, label it "Activity 8-5," and place it in your assignment folder.**

8. Close out of the *Statement* by clicking on the "X" in the upper-right-hand corner.

Activity 8-6

View and Reprint a Patient Statement Using the Financial Module

The *Statements* application in the *Financial* module (**Figure 8-32**) allows you to view and reprint statements that have been generated for the patient in context. A statement can be reprinted by clicking on the *Print View* button next to the appropriate statement line. When *Print View* is clicked, the patient's statement displays in a new window, and by right-clicking on top of it, the statement can be printed.

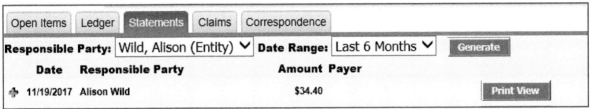

Figure 8-32   Statements Application in Financial Module

Courtesy of Harris Care Tracker PM and EMR

1. Pull patient Alison Wild into context.

2. Click the *Financial* module. Click *Go*. The *Open Items* for the patient display (**Figure 8-33**). (**Note:** You can also access the open items by clicking the *OI* icon on the *Name Bar*.)

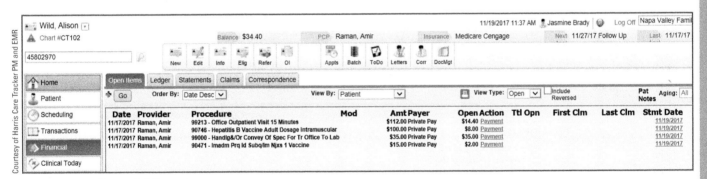

Figure 8-33   Financial Open Items

3. Click the *Statements* tab. Harris CareTracker PM opens the *Statements* application (see **Figure 8-34**).

   a. The *Responsible Party* list defaults to the responsible party set in the patient's demographic. Leave as is. (**Note:** You can select a different responsible party or "(All)" responsible parties, if applicable.)

   b. The *Date Range* list defaults to "Last 6 Months." Use the drop-down next to *Date Range* and select "All Dates."

4. Click *Generate*. Harris CareTracker PM generates a list of the patient's statements and displays a processing message in the lower frame of the screen.

5. Select the *Click Here* link in blue (noted in Figure 8-34). The application displays the list of statements.

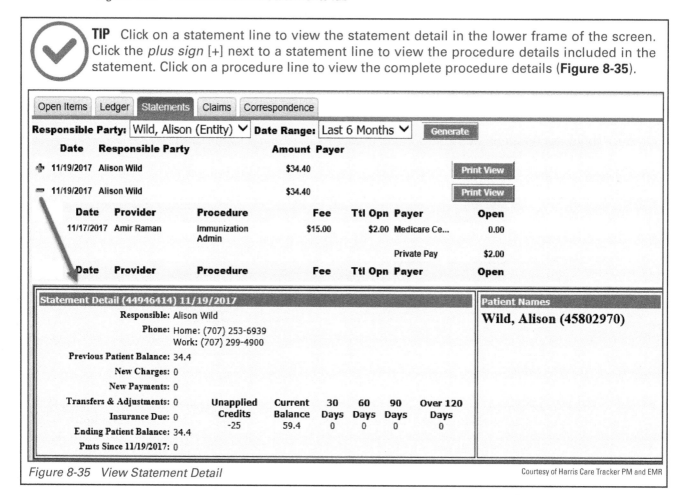

Figure 8-34   Financial Module/Statements Tab

✓ **TIP** Click on a statement line to view the statement detail in the lower frame of the screen. Click the *plus sign* [+] next to a statement line to view the procedure details included in the statement. Click on a procedure line to view the complete procedure details (**Figure 8-35**).

Figure 8-35   View Statement Detail

6. Click *Print View* next to the statement you want to print. Select the most recent statement. The application displays the statement in a new window. **Note:** It may take a few moments to display.

7. Right-click on the statement and then select *Print* from the shortcut menu or click on the *Print* icon in the upper-right corner.

🖶 **Print the statement, label it "Activity 8-6," and place it in your assignment folder.**

8. Close the statement window when the statement has printed.

PATIENT COLLECTIONS

Learning Objective 4: Review collection status and transfer private pay balances.

Activity 8-7

Transfer a Balance

The *Collections* application in Harris CareTracker PM allows you to focus collection efforts on patients with balances at least 30 days overdue. You can determine whether patients are identified by the collections system immediately or after their balance is 30, 60, 90, or 120 days overdue.

A patient balance will automatically appear in *Collections* when the balance ages past the days set in *Days Overdue* and one additional statement has generated. When "Immediate" is selected, the system will send a patient directly to the *Collections* module after his or her first statement is generated. The collections' setting applies to all groups in the company.

All new patients added to the *Collections* application will have a collection status of "New" and should be reviewed weekly to determine if they should be removed from *Collections* or if some type of collection action should be taken. However, when the patient balance reaches zero, Harris CareTracker PM automatically removes the patient from the *Collections* list.

> **TIP** To verify whether the patient qualifies for *Collections*, click the *Statements* tab in the *Financial* module. Click on the most recent statement and review the aging in the *Statement Detail* (**Figure 8-36**). If the aging has not met the *Days Overdue* setting, the patient will not appear in *Collections*.

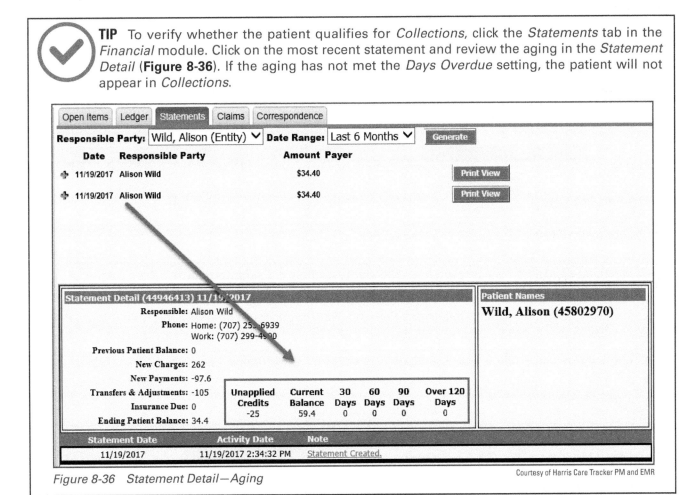

Figure 8-36   Statement Detail—Aging

Courtesy of Harris Care Tracker PM and EMR

In addition to managing the balance transfers, when you send a patient's balance to a collection agency, you should change his or her patient status to *Collections*. This can be done in the *Demographics* application by selecting "Collections" from the *Category* drop-down list (**Figure 8-37**). This status will always display next to the patient's name in Harris CareTracker PM (**Figure 8-38**) so all staff will know that this patient has been transferred to the collection agency. For the *Collections* notice to appear, you will have to take the patient out of context and then bring back into context before *Collections* status appears.

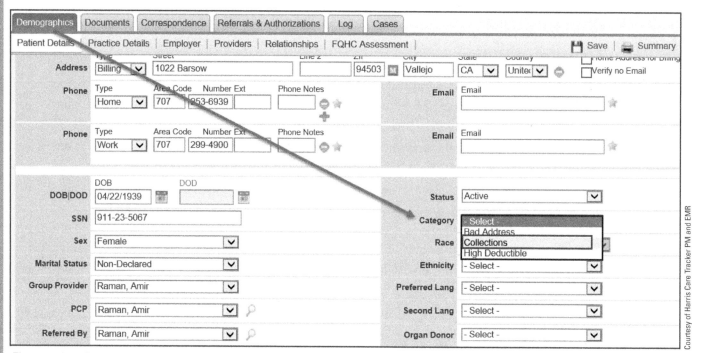

Figure 8-37   Patient Category—Collections in Demographics Screen

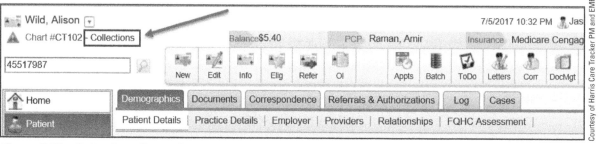

Figure 8-38   Collections Status Appears Next to Chart Number

The *Collections* application is accessed from the *Home* module > *Dashboard* tab > *Billing* section > *Collections* link (**Figure 8-39**). There are seven collection statuses in Harris CareTracker PM: New, Open Collections, Review, Collections Actual, Collections Pending, Collections Pending – NS, and Hold (**Figure 8-40**).

 TIP   You must have a batch open to transfer any balances from private pay to *Collect Pend Statement*.

Moving Patients to Collections

Harris CareTracker PM automatically moves patients into *Collections* when their overdue balance reaches the aging level assigned in the group settings and automatically removes patients from *Collections* when their overdue balance is paid. Operators can also move patients in and out of *Collections* manually. In

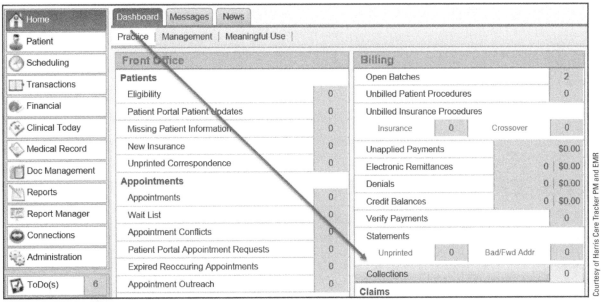

Figure 8-39   Collections Link

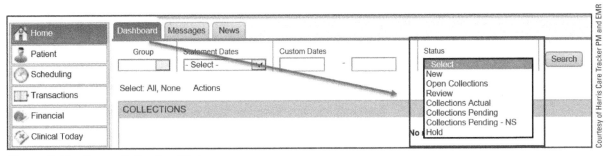

Figure 8-40   Seven Collection Statuses

Open Items, you can add a patient to *Collections* by clicking the *Add Responsible Party* link in the *Collections* work area or by transferring a balance to *Collections*.

Patients manually added to *Collections* are flagged with an asterisk (*) next to their name in the work area. Patients manually added to *Collections* must be removed from *Collections* manually as well. When manually adding a patient to *Collections*, Harris CareTracker PM pulls the patient into context and filters the *Collections* list to show the responsible party for that patient.

To Transfer a Balance:

1. Go to the *Home* module > *Dashboard* tab > *Billing* section > *Collections* link. Harris CareTracker PM displays a list of collection statuses and the number of patients in each status.

2. If there is no patient listed, click the *Add Responsible Party* link in the upper-right corner of the screen.

3. In the *Add Manual Collection* window, click the *Search* icon and enter the name of the patient you are searching for (select patient Alison Wild). Click on the patient name in the *Results* window. The patient name now populates in the *Add Manual Collection* window.

4. Click *Save*.

5. Click the *Edit* icon next to the balance you want to transfer to a new financial class. Harris CareTracker PM displays the *Edit* window (**Figure 8-41**).

   a. *Insurance*: Leave blank (-Select-).

   b. *Overdue*: Leave blank (-Select-).

   c. *Letter*: Leave blank (-Select-).

   d. *Change Status*: Select "Open Collections."

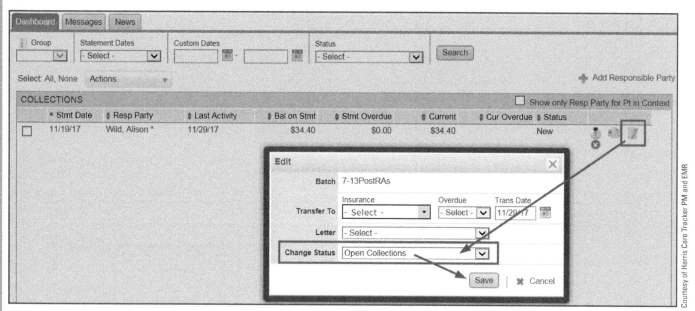

Figure 8-41   Edit Collections Dialog Box

6. Click *Save*.

7. In the *Updates Processed* window that appears, click *Close*. Harris CareTracker PM updates the patient's status in the *Collections* application, transfers the outstanding balance to the selected financial class, and adds the selected "Transfer To" financial class to the patient's *Demographics* record.

TIP To transfer multiple balances to a new financial class, select the checkbox next to each balance you want to transfer and then click *Actions > Edit* (**Figure 8-42**).

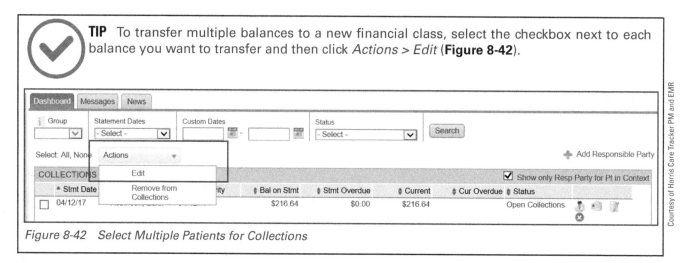

Figure 8-42   Select Multiple Patients for Collections

Print the Balance Transfer screen, label it "Activity 8-7," and place it in your assignment folder.

You can add the *Collections Pending Statement, Collections Pending No Statement, Collections Actual* financial classes, or your collection agency name to the *Insurance Plans* "quick picks" list in the *Quick Picks* application in the *Administration* module.

COLLECTION LETTERS

Learning Objective 5: Create collection letters.

PROFESSIONALISM CONNECTION

Collection letters should do two things: retain customer goodwill and help you get paid. One way to know if the letter is working is based on the response received. A good letter will generate multiple responses (phone calls and/or payments). If you send a batch of letters and there is no response, it may be time to revise your collection letters and/or procedure. Any correspondence from the medical office is a reflection of the practice, so keep it professional.

Your letter is intended to persuade someone to send you money; therefore, the wording and tone are critical, especially if this is a patient you want to continue to do business with. Enclosing an envelope for payment is always a good idea. If you can include postage on the payment envelope, that is even better. The easier you make it for the customer to make the payment, the better your chances are of getting paid. If you cannot include a pre-paid return envelope (due to high cost), propose an alternative form of payment (i.e., credit/debit card). Always remember to close the letter with an appropriate salutation.

Review the "Global Collection Letters" available in the templates provided and see if they fit with the "message" you want to send to the patient along with the appropriate "image" of the practice. How would you feel if you received one of the generic "collections" letter? How could you customize the language to accomplish the goal of collecting money due, yet keeping the relationship with the patient intact?

 ## Activity 8-8
Create a Custom Collection Letter

The *Global Collection Letters* application contains the following letters, which are available to all users in Harris CareTracker PM.

- "Collections 1": Explains that the account is overdue and lists the overdue balance.

- "Past Due": Explains that the overdue balance or a portion of the balance is more than 60 days past due.

- "Delinquent": Explains that the overdue balance or a portion of the balance is more than 90 days past due.

- "Final Notice": Tells the patient that her overdue balance or a portion of her balance is more than 120 days past due. This is the final written notice the patient will receive, and, if payment is not received, the account will be sent to *Collections*.

- "75 Collection": States that if the overdue balance is not paid in full, the billing office will continue with its collection policy, which may include using a collection agency.

- "Collection Payment Plan": Informs the patient that she can set up a weekly or monthly payment plan to pay off the overdue balance. On a "Collection Payment Plan" letter, the patient can also indicate if she has insurance that covered the services for which she has an overdue balance. When a patient indicates that he or she has insurance to cover the services, the patient must also complete the insurance section on the back of a statement.

You can also create custom collection letters in the *Letter Editor* application in the *Administration* module.

When you create a group-specific collection letter, the top portion of the letter by default includes patient information, such as name, address, and so on. The only portion of the letter you need to build in the *Letter Editor* is the text you want to appear in the letter.

Group-specific collection letters are built in the *Practice Letter Editor* in the *Administration* module. After creating a custom collection letter, you must add the letter to your *Form Letters Quick Picks* via the *Quick Picks* application in the *Administration* module. This will allow you to access the letter in the *Collections* module.

To Create a Custom Collection Letter:

1. Go to the *Administration* module > *Practice* tab > *Forms and Letters* section > *Practice Letter Editor* link (**Figure 8-43**).

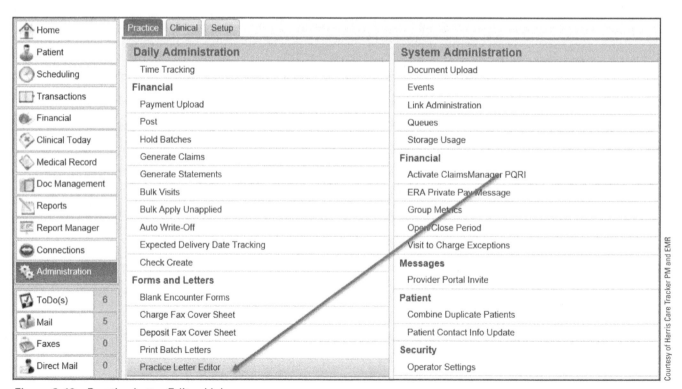

Figure 8-43   *Practice Letter Editor Link*

2. From the *Letters* drop-down list, select "Create New Letter" (**Figure 8-44**). The application displays the *New Letter* window (**Figure 8-45**).

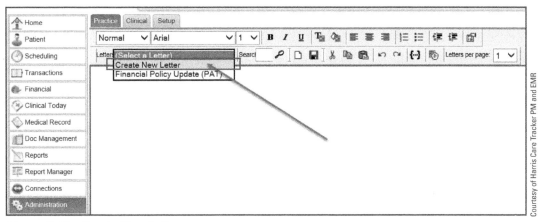

Figure 8-44   Create New Letter

3. Enter a descriptive name for the form letter in the *Letter Name* field. Enter "Missed Appointment Fee."

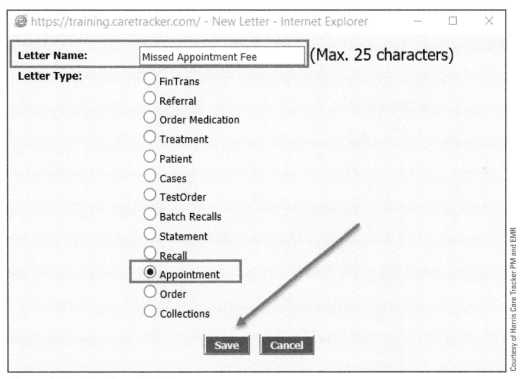

Figure 8-45   New Letter Window

4. In the *Letter Type* field, select the radio button next to the type of form letter you are creating (select "Appointment").

5. Then click *Save* (see Figure 8-51). The application closes the *New Letter* window and pulls the new letter name and type into the *Letters* field (**Figure 8-46**). **Note:** It may take a few moments for the screen to refresh.

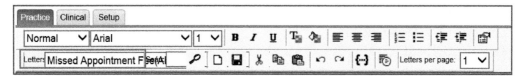

Figure 8-46   Letters Field

6. Enter the text to appear in the form letter and insert data fields where necessary using the *Select Field* {⋯} icon. Select data fields from the drop-down list in the *Select Field* list (**Figure 8-47**) to complete your letter. (For example, for the first line of the letter, select "Current Date - Long" from the *Special Fields* section in the *Select Field* list.) As a best practice, you should click *Save* 🖫 icon periodically while building your letter. Be sure to format the letter as you would like it to appear, following the instructions below:

    a. Click on the *Select Field* icon, scroll down to the *Special Fields* section, and select "Current Date – Long," then click [enter] to move the line. Recall that the *Letter Editor* is preset to double space when you hit the [Enter] key to enter a new line of text. For single spacing, hold the [Shift] key down as you press the [Enter] key.

    b. Click on the *Select Field* icon, scroll down, and in the *Patient Fields (General)* select "First Name."

    c. Staying on the same line, click on the *Select Field* icon, scroll down, and in the *Patient Fields (General)* select "Last Name."

    d. Staying on the same line, click on the *Select Field* icon, scroll down, and in the *Patient Fields (Billing Address)* select "Address 1."

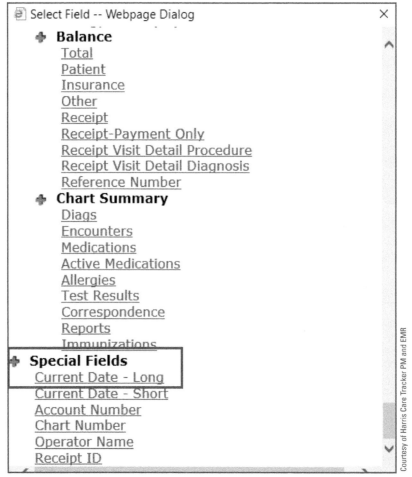

Figure 8-47   Select Field List

e. Staying on the same line, click on the *Select Field* icon, scroll down, and in the *Patient Fields (Billing Address)* select "City."

f. Staying on the same line, click on the *Select Field* icon, scroll down, and in the *Patient Fields (Billing Address)* select "State Code."

g. Staying on the same line, click on the *Select Field* icon, scroll down, and in the *Patient Fields (Billing Address)* select "Zip Code."

h. Hit [Enter] to move to the next line.

i. Type "Dear", then a space.

j. Then staying on the same line, click on the *Select Field* icon, scroll down, and in the *Patient Fields (General)* select "Title."

k. Staying on the same line, click on the *Select Field* icon, scroll down, and in the *Patient Fields (General)* select "Last Name."

l. Hit [Enter] to move to the next line.

m. Type in the following message:

"You missed your last scheduled appointment with Dr. [(click on the *Select Field* icon, scroll down, and in the *Primary Care Provider (PCP)* field select "Last Name"] on [click on the *Select Field* icon, scroll down, and in the *Appointment* field select "Date Only"]. We are concerned about your health and would like to reschedule the appointment at your earliest convenience. There is a $35 charge for appointments that are canceled with less than 8-business hours' notice. Please remit to our billing office.

Please call the office to schedule or select an appointment via the Patient Portal.

If you have any questions, please don't hesitate to call.

Sincerely,

Jasmine Brady, MA, Office Manager"

n. Your screen should look like **Figure 8-48**.

7. Click the *Save File* 💾 icon when you are finished with your form letter.

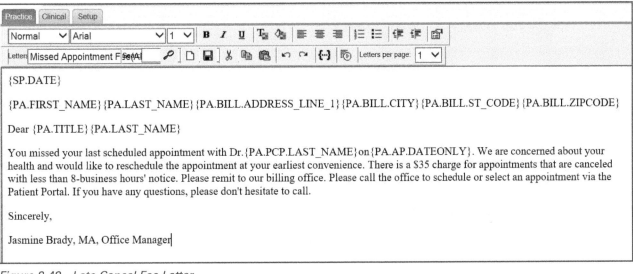

Figure 8-48   Late Cancel Fee Letter

Print the screen that displays the Custom Collection Letter, label it "Activity 8-8," and place it in your assignment folder.

Activity 8-9
Add a Form Letter to Quick Picks

After creating a new form letter, you must add it to your *Quick Picks* to make it available for use in Harris CareTracker PM and EMR.

1. Go to the *Administration* module > *Setup* tab > *Financial* section > *Quick Picks* link.

2. From the *Screen Type* drop-down list, select "Form Letters" (**Figure 8-49**).

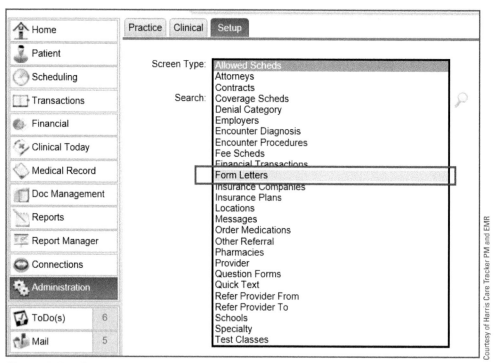

Figure 8-49   *Screen Type—Form Letters*

3. In the *Search* field, enter part of the name of the new form letter you created in Activity 8-8 (enter "Missed") and then click the *Search* 🔍 icon. The application displays a pop-up of all of the letters that match the search criteria (**Figure 8-50**).

4. Click on the form letter you want to add to your *Quick Picks* list (select "Missed Appointment Fee"). You will receive a pop-up *Success* box stating "Quick Pick information has been updated."

5. Click *Close* on the *Success* box (**Figure 8-51**).

6. The application adds the letter to the *Quick Picks* list where it will be available to generate for patients.

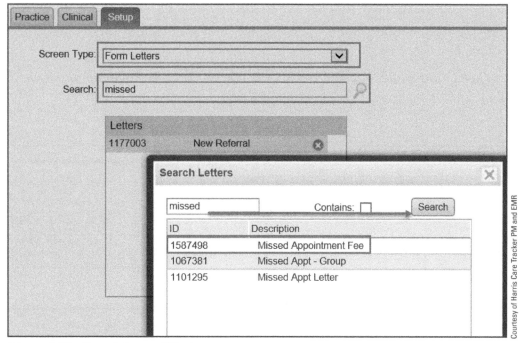

Figure 8-50   Search Letters Window

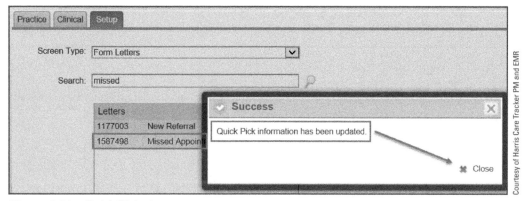

Figure 8-51   Quick Picks Letters

Print the Quick Picks list screen with the Form Letter added, label it "Activity 8-9," and place it in your assignment folder.

GENERATE COLLECTION LETTERS

Learning Objective 6: Generate collection letters.

Activity 8-10
Generate Collection Letters

To generate collection letters, use one of two options: Harris CareTracker PM and EMR's global collection letters, or build a custom collection letter specific to your practice. After collection letters have been generated, they must be printed from the *Print Batch Letters* application in the *Administration* module. Generated collection letters are saved in the patients' record in the *Correspondence* application of the *Financial* module.

1. Go to the *Home* module > *Dashboard* tab > *Billing* section > *Collections* link. Harris CareTracker PM displays a list of collection statements (**Figure 8-52**).

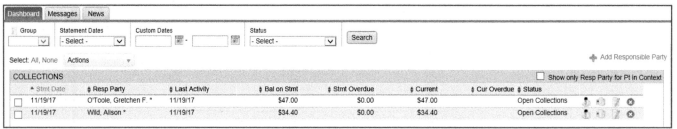

Figure 8-52 Search Collections Fields

2. Use the filters at the top of the page to view statements by *Group, Status,* or date range. For this activity, in the drop-down list in the *Status* field, leave as (-Select-) and click *Search* (**Figure 8-53**).

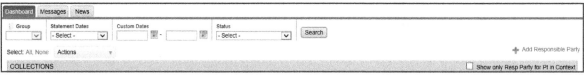

Figure 8-53 Search Collections Results

3. Double-click the name "Alison Wild" in the line of the *Responsible Party* column to view the *Statement Details* (**Figure 8-54**). It is helpful to review this information when determining a status change and/or deciding what action to take on a patient's balance.

4. Close out of the *Statement Detail* dialog box.

5. Click the *Edit* icon next to the statement line for which you want to generate a collection letter (Alison Wild). Harris CareTracker PM displays the *Edit* box.

6. From the *Letter* list, select the letter you want to generate. Select "Past Due 60 1st" (**Figure 8-55**).

7. If needed, select a new status from the *Change Status* list. (Leave blank: "-Select-".)

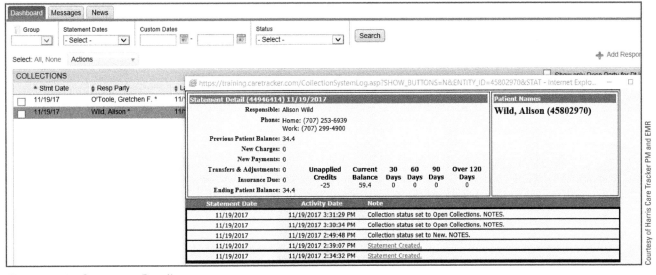

Figure 8-54   Statement Details

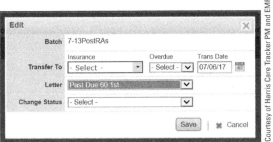

Figure 8-55   Generate Past Due 60 1st Letter

 TIP To generate letters for multiple patients, select the checkbox next to each patient for whom you want to generate a letter and then click *Actions > Edit*.

Print the Edit window, label it "Activity 8-10," and place it in your assignment folder.

8. Click *Save.*

9. Then close out of the *Updates Processed* window. Generated collection letters can be printed from the *Print Batch Letters* application in the *Administration* module (**Figure 8-56**). You will receive an error message because you are not able to print batch letters in your student version of Harris CareTracker.

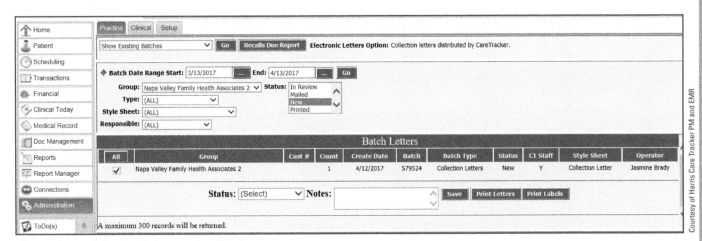

Figure 8-56   Print Batch Letters Application

FYI If you do not print the collection letters, in a live environment, Harris CareTracker PM and EMR will automatically print the letters to send out to the patient the next day.

Activity 8-11
Run a Journal and Post All Remaining Batches

1. Go to the *Reports* module > *Todays Journals* link.

2. Click on *Add All>>.*

3. Scroll down and place a check mark in the *Includes Transfers* checkbox.

4. Click *Create Journal.*

🖬 **Print the Journal, label it "Activity 8-11a," and place it in your assignment folder.**

5. Go to the *Home* module > *Dashboard* tab > *Billing* section > *Open Batches* link. Harris CareTracker PM displays a list of open batches.

6. Place a check mark in the *Batch Name* column by each unposted batch.

🖬 **Print the Batches to Post screen, label it "Activity 8-11b," and place it in your assignment folder.**

7. Click *Post Batches.*

CRITICAL THINKING Billing and collections activities require the utmost professionalism. Having completed your studies and activities in this chapter, do you feel more (or less) comfortable working collections? How would you apply professionalism skills to the situation where a patient desperately needs medical care and medication, but cannot afford either? How would you deal with an angry patient when you need to discuss finances? Can you think of ways to avoid difficult situations with patients and billing and collections? Consider also how the practice is affected by your ability to collect fees due.

If you have had the opportunity to role-play with your fellow students or a family member with various collection scenarios, did that help with preparedness, conveying empathy, and noting the tone and inflection in your voice? Share your experiences with your instructor and classmates.

CASE STUDIES

For patient Alec Winfrey, complete the following activities:

Case Study 8-1

Generate a statement. (Refer to Activity 8-5 for guidance.)

(**Note**: If statement is not displaying after you complete the steps or you receive an error message, click back on the *Administration* module, *Generate Statements* link and repeat the steps.)

🖬 **Print the Generated Statement, label it "Case Study 8-1," and place it in your assignment folder.**

(*continues*)

(*continued*)

Case Study 8-2

Transfer any remaining balance to *Open Collections* for Alec Winfrey. See Activity 10-7 for guidance. Note that you will need to click *Add Responsible Party* and add the patient in order for Alec Winfrey to appear in the *Add Manual Collection* window.

🖳 **Once balance has been transferred, print the screen showing the Transferred Balance, label it "Case Study 8-2," and place it in your assignment folder.**

Case Study 8-3

Generate collection letter (Past Due 60 1st) for patient Alec Winfrey. Once the patient has had the collections letter generated, click on the *Correspondence* 🔖 icon after *Status* "Open Collections" for the patient. The *Patient Correspondence* dialog box displays. Print the *Correspondence Log* for the patient.

🖳 **Print the Correspondence Log showing the Collection Letters generated for the patient, label it "Case Study 8-3," and place it in your assignment folder.**

Applied Learning for the Paperless Medical Office

Learning Objectives

1. Perform EMR tasks related to registering and scheduling a patient, completing the visit, billing the appointment, and collecting payment.

INTRODUCTION

Congratulations on completing the activities in Chapters 1 through 8! You will now apply what you learned to the case studies in this chapter. Completing these case studies will help you increase your proficiency in a real-world electronic health record.

If you need help completing these case studies, a guide has been posted to the student companion website. This guide references activities within this book that you can review for assistance.

> Before you begin the activities in this chapter, refresh your memory on working with Harris CareTracker by referring back to the Best Practices list on page xiv of this workbook. This list is also posted to the student companion website. Following best practices will help you complete work quickly and accurately.

CASE STUDY 9-1: GRETCHEN O'TOOLE

Gretchen O'Toole is an established patient who calls the office this morning to schedule an appointment with Dr. Brockton, her primary care provider. She says she wants to see Dr. Brockton regarding her diabetes management because she has not been feeling well the past few weeks. Gretchen has not been in to see Dr. Brockton since the office converted to electronic records, but she is registered in the database. Search the database confirming her DOB, current address, phone number, and insurance, and then schedule the appointment for her.

Step 1: Search the Database and Schedule an Appointment

1. Search the database for patient Gretchen O'Toole. Update her demographics to include Dr. Brockton as her PCP, and change her *Consent* and *NPP* to "Yes."

2. Schedule an appointment for Gretchen with Dr. Brockton, using the first available morning slot, or by double-booking the 11:00 a.m. slot. (**Note**: If you are entering data on a weekend, or a day when there is no availability in the schedule, select an appointment day on the first <u>prior</u> date available. This will ensure you can complete activities by not working in a "future date."

- *Appointment Type*: Follow Up
- *Complaint*: Diabetes Management
- *Location*: NVFA

Step 2: Check In Patient

1. When Gretchen arrives for her appointment, view her *At-A-Glance* (*Info*) patient information to confirm that she is still insured with Century Med PPO and has a $35.00 copay.

2. Before accepting Gretchen's payment, create a new batch named "OTooleCS."

3. Accept and enter Gretchen's cash payment for her copay and print a receipt for her.

Label the printed receipt "Case Study 9-1A."

4. Check Gretchen in for her visit with Dr. Brockton.

Step 3: Patient Work-Up

To begin EMR activities, edit your operator preferences for clinical workflows in your batch with Dr. Brockton as the provider.

Background Information about Gretchen O'Toole

Gretchen was diagnosed with type 2 diabetes mellitus approximately 20 years ago—around the same time she was diagnosed with hypertension. She has been very compliant over the years and remains on an oral hypoglycemic. She is here for a routine follow-up appointment exam after discovering at a local church health fair that her cholesterol is elevated and wants to discuss the findings with the doctor.

1. Accessing the patient's chart through *Clinical Today*, *transfer* Gretchen to Exam Room #1.

2. Ms. O'Toole is being seen today for diabetes management and hypertension. Because Gretchen is now ready to see Dr. Brockton, create a progress note for her. Refer to **Table 9-1** while completing the progress note. Select progress note template "IM OV Option 4 (v4) w/A&P." (**Note**: You will be acting as a scribe for the provider in this case study, meaning you will free text much of the medical record information in the *Progress Note*.)

When you have completed Step 3: Patient Work-up, print the patient's Chart Summary, and label it "Case Study 9-1B."

Completing the Visit by Entering Lab Orders

Before Gretchen leaves the office, the clinical medical assistant will add a *Recall* for her CPE one year plus one day from today's date, and complete the *Orders* and *Referral* in the *Plan* section of the progress note. As the biller and coder, you will not be entering the lab orders, recall, or referral and will instead move on to capturing the visit.

Table 9-1   Gretchen O'Toole Progress Note Information

TAB	ENTRY
CC/HPI	*Chief Complaint:* Select "Established Patient" and "Follow-Up Visit" boxes.
	Other complaints box: Free text "Wants cholesterol checked. Had blood test (finger stick) at a church health fair. Result was elevated. Does not recall reading."
	History of Present Illness box: Free text "Pt. here for a F/U exam for diabetes and hypertension. Pt. states she checks her blood sugar in the morning when she first gets up and 2 hours after each meal. 'Readings have stayed below 130 mg/dL.' Last A1c was in October of last year, result 6.4. Pt. also states that home blood pressure readings have been running between 140 and 160 on the systolic side and between 85 and 95 on the diastolic side. Pt. has some tingling in her toes but not often. Regularly sees an ophthamologist for eye care. Overall, pt. states that she feels very good!"
Skip the HX, ROS, PE, TESTS, and PROC Tabs	(No entry)
ASSESS	*Diagnoses:* Autonomic neuropathy in diseases classified elsewhere (G99.0); Essential (primary) hypertension (I10); Type 2 diabetes mellitus with other diabetic neurological complication (E11.49); Overweight (E66.3)
PLAN	*Additional Plan Details* box—free-text the following: 1. EKG 2. Hemoglobin A1c/Hemoglobin total in blood 3. Glucose Blood Test—Global 4. Lipid panel with direct LDL in serum or plasma 5. Have patient follow up with podiatrist; Referrl to Dr. William R. Todd, DPM in Napa, CA 6. Rx: MetFORMIN HCl Oral Tablet 850 mg. Sig: One 850 mg tablet twice a day, 180 tabs. 4 refills 7. Rx: Micardis Oral Tablet 40 mg. Sig: One 40 mg tablet daily, 90 tabs, 4 refills, take in the evening 8. Patient Education Materials: PERIPHERAL NEUROPATHY HIGH BLOOD PRESSURE-ESTABLISHED 9. 3-month follow-up appointment 10. Referral to Podiatrist: Dr. William R. Todd, DPM in Napa, CA

*Remember to *Save* the progress note.

Step 4: Capture the Visit and Sign the Note

Now that all of the orders as indicated in the progress note are completed, capture the *Visit* and sign the progress note (review the A&P to be sure you captured all billable items).

1. Capture the *Visit* by entering:

   - In the *Procedures* tab, enter CPT® *code(s)*: 99213; 82962; 80061; 36415; 93000; and 99000

     Source: Current Procedural Terminology © 2017 American Medical Association.

   - In the *Diagnosis* tab, enter *ICD-10 code(s)*: E11.49; G99.0, I10; and E66.3

2. Sign the progress note.

📇 **Print the signed progress note and label it "Case Study 9-1C."**

3. Before Gretchen leaves, schedule her follow-up appointment noted in the *Plan* section of the progress note.

Step 5: Verify Charges

Verify charges for Gretchen's *Visit* and then generate a claim.

1. Using the batch you created at the beginning of the case study, run a journal and verify charges.

📇 **Print the Journal and label it "Case Study 9-1D."**

Step 6: Process Remittance (EOB/RA) and Transfer to Private Pay

1. Save the charges for the visit for Ms. O'Toole. (**Hint:** Check your batch and make sure you are working in the batch "OTooleCS." If not, edit the batch and using the drop-downs, select the parameters as set in the original batch.

2. Build all claims for Gretchen's visit.

3. Refer to Gretchen's EOB/RA (Source Document 9-1 at the end of this case study) and process the remittance.

4. Run a journal to verify charges.

📇 **Print the journal and label it "Case Study 9-1E."**

Step 7: Work Claims and Generate Patient Statement

1. Work the *Claims Worklist.*

2. Post all open batches.

3. Generate a statement for Gretchen.

📇 **Print the statement and label it "Case Study 9-1F."**

CASE STUDY 9-2: TRANSFER TO COLLECTIONS

Scenario: It has now been more than 60 days since you generated a statement for Gretchen and her payment has not been received.

1. Manually transfer Gretchen's account to *Open Collections.*

2. Generate a collection letter appropriate to the office policy for accounts older than 60 days.

📇 **Print a screenshot of the Collections screen listing these outstanding accounts and label it "Case Study 9-2."**

Source Document 9-1:   Explanation of Benefits/Remittance Advice

CENTURY CENGAGE

CENTURY CENGAGE
P.O. Box 87542
San Jose, CA 95101

Date: MM/DD/YYYY (Appt. date used in Case Study 9-1)
Payment Number: 2344570
Payment Amount: $148.94

ANTHONY BROCKTON, M.D.
Napa Valley Family Health Associates (NVFHA)
101 Vine Street
Napa, CA 94558

Account Number	Patient Name				Subscriber Number		Claim Number			
Dates of Service	Description of Service	Amount Charged	Not Covered (DENIAL)	Prov Adj Discount	Amount Allowed	Deduct/Coins/Copay	Paid to Provider	Adj Reason Code	Rmk Code	Patient Resp
9706416	O'Toole, Gretchen									
(Appt. date used in Case Study 9-1)	99213	$112.00		$0.00	$112.00	$35.00	$77.00	45*		$0.00
(Appt. date used in Case Study 9-1)	99000	$35.00		$25.00	$10.00	$2.00	$8.00	20*		$2.00
(Appt. date used in Case Study 9-1)	82962	$10.00		$0.00	$10.00	$5.00	$5.00	45*		$5.00
(Appt. date used in Case Study 9-1)	80061	$37.44		$0.00	$37.44	$20.00	$17.44	45*		$20.00
(Appt. date used in Case Study 9-1)	36415	$15.00		$0.00	$15.00	$5.00	$10.00	45*		$5.00
(Appt. date used in Case Study 9-1)	93000	$46.50		$0.00	$46.50	$15.00	$31.50	45*		$15.00
TOTALS		$255.94		$25.00	$230.94	$82.00	$148.94			$47.00

Amount Allowed (45*) = Charges exceed your contracted/legislated fee arrangement
Amount Allowed (20*) = Not a covered code

Resources

ABC News.com. (2009, July 16). *President Obama continues questionable "You Can Keep Your Health Care" promise*. Retrieved from http://abcnews.go.com/blogs/politics/2009/07/president-obama- continues-questionable-you-can-keep-your-health-care-promise/

American Academy of Family Physicians. (2003). The HIPAA privacy rules: three key forms. Retrieved from http://www.aafp.org/fpm/2003/0200/p29.html

American Association of Professional Coders (AAPC). https://www.aapc.com/

American Medical Association (AMA). https://www.ama-assn.org

Bureau of Labor Statistics, U.S. Department of Labor. (2014). *Occupational Outlook Handbook*. Medical Records and Health Information Technicians. Retrieved from http://www.bls.gov/ooh/healthcare/medical-records-and-health-information-technicians.htm

Centers for Medicare and Medicaid Services. (n.d.). Retrieved from http://www.cms.gov/Regulations-and-Guidance/HIPAA-Administrative-Simplification/Versions5010andD0/index.html

Centers for Medicare and Medicaid Services. (n.d.). Delivery system reform, medicare payment reform. Retrieved from https://www.cms.gov/Medicare/Quality-Initiatives-Patient-Assessment-Instruments/Value-Based-Programs/MACRA-MIPS-and-APMs/MACRA-MIPS-and-APMs.html

Centers for Medicare and Medicaid Services (CMS). (n.d.). Glossary. Retrieved from the CMS website http://www.medicare.gov/glossary/f.html

Centers for Medicare and Medicaid Services. (n.d.). *Meaningful use*. Retrieved from http://www.cms.gov/Regulations-and-Guidance/Legislation/EHRIncentivePrograms/Meaningful_Use.html

CertMedAssistants.com. (n.d.). Retrieved from http://www.certmedassistant.com/

Coding classification standards. (n.d.). Retrieved from www.ahima.org

Department of Health and Human Services (DHHS), *Centers for Medicare and Medicaid Services (CMS).* (2003, June 6). Medicare hospital manual. Retrieved from http://www.cms.gov/Regulations-and-Guidance/Guidance/Transmittals/downloads/R804HO.pdf

Department of Health and Human Services (DHHS), Centers for Medicare and Medicaid (CMS). (n.d.). Remittance advice information: an overview. Fact sheet. Retrieved from https://www.cms.gov/Outreach-and-Education/Medicare-Learning-Network-MLN/MLNProducts/Downloads/Remit-Advice-Overview-Fact-Sheet-ICN908325.pdf

Duke Clinical Research Institute. (n.d.). Beers criteria medication list. Retrieved from https://www.dcri.org/beers-criteria-medication-list/

General information: Nurse practitioner practice. (2011, April 13). Retrieved from http://www.rn.ca.gov/pdfs/regulations/npr-b-23.pdf

Health Information and Management Systems Society. (2008, August). *Real time adjudication of healthcare claims* (HIMSS Financial Systems Financial Transactions Toolkit Task Force White Paper). Retrieved from http://himss.files.cms-plus.com/HIMSSorg/content/files/Line%2027%20-%20Real%20Time%20Adjudication%20of%20Healthcare%20Claims.pdf

Health Information Technology for Economic and Clinical Health (HITECH). (2013, November 27). HITECH Act Enforcement Interim Final Rule.

HealthIT.gov. (n.d.). *EHR incentives and certification.* Retrieved from https://www.healthit.gov/providers-professionals/ehr-incentive-payment-timeline

HealthIT.gov. (n.d.). Meaningful use definitions and objectives. Retrieved from https://www.healthit.gov/providers-professionals/meaningful-use-definition-objectives

HealthIT.gov. (n.d.). What does "interoperability" mean and why is it important. Retrieved from https://www.healthit.gov/providers-professionals/faqs/what-does-interoperability-mean-and-why-it-important

HealthIT.gov. (n.d.). What is meaningful use? Retrieved from http://www.healthit.gov/policy-researchers-implementers/meaningful-use

HealthIT.gov. (2013, January). Are there penalties for providers who don't switch to electronic health records (EHR)? Retrieved from https://www.healthit.gov/providers-professionals/faqs/are-there-penalties-providers-who-don%E2%80%99t-switch-electronic-health-record

Health Resources and Services Administration (of the HHS). (n.d.). Retrieved from http://www.hrsa.gov/index.html

Indian Health Service. (n.d.). Medicare and Medicaid incentives for EPs. Retrieved from https://www.ihs.gov/meaningfuluse/incentivesoverview/incentivesep/

Institute for Healthcare Improvement. (n.d.). The five rights of medication administration. Retrieved from http://www.ihi.org/resources/pages/improvementstories/fiverightsofmedicationadministration.aspx

Institute of Medicine of the National Academies. (2003, July 31). *Key capabilities of an electronic health record system.* Retrieved from http://www.iom.edu/Reports/2003/Key-Capabilities-of-an-Electronic-Health-Record-System.aspx

Internal Revenue Service. (2016, November). Questions and Answers about Reporting Social Security Numbers to Your Health Insurance Company. Retrieved from https://www.irs.gov/affordable-care-act/questions-and-answers-about-reporting-social-security-numbers-to-your-health-insurance-company.

Kaiser Family Foundation. (2016, September). Key facts about the uninsured population. Retrieved from http://kff.org/uninsured/fact-sheet/key-facts-about-the-uninsured-population/

Lowes, Robert. (2015, August). e-Prescribing controlled substances now legal nationwide. Retrieved from http://www.medscape.com/viewarticle/850268

"Meaningful Use." *Centers for Medicare and Medicaid Services.* (2014, February 8). Retrieved from http://www .cms.gov/Regulations-and-Guidance/Legislation/EHRIncentivePrograms/Meaningful_Use.html.

Medicare.gov. (n.d.). Your medicare coverage. Is my test, item, or service covered? Retrieved from https://www.medicare.gov/coverage/cervical-vaginal-cancer-screenings.html

Menachemi, N., & Collum, T. H. (2011). Benefits and drawbacks of electronic health record systems. *Risk Management and Healthcare Policy*, 4, 47–55. Retrieved from http://www .ncbi.nlm.nih.gov/pmc/articles/PMC3270933/

National Healthcareer Association. (n.d.). *Certified electronic health records specialist (CEHRS™).* Retrieved from http://www.nhanow.com/health-record.aspx

New Health Advisor. (2016). 10 rights of medication administration. http://www.newhealthadvisor.com/10-Rights-of-Medication-Administration.html

Rowley, R. (2011). *Ambulatory vs. hospital EHRs.* Retrieved from http://www.practicefusion.com/ehrbloggers/2011/07/ambulatory-vs-hospital-ehrs.html

SNOMED Overview: Clinical Terms and SNOMED Terminology Solutions. (2008, July 3). Retrieved from /files/HIMSSorg/content/files/snomed_101overview.pdf

The American Health Quality Association, Quality Update. (2003, August 22). Retrieved from www.ahqa.org

The Fiscal Times. (2016, May). Even with obamacare, 29 million people are uninsured; here's why. Retrieved from http://www.thefiscaltimes.com/2016/05/10/Even-Obamacare-29-Million-People-Are-Uninsured-Here-s-Why

U.S. Department of Commerce, U.S. Census Bureau, American National Standards Institute. (2013). Retrieved from http://www.census.gov/geo/www/ansi/ansi.html

U.S. Department of Health and Human Services. (n.d.). *HIPAA for Individuals.* Retrieved from http://www.hhs.gov/hipaa/for-individuals/index.html.

U.S. Department of Health and Human Services. (n.d.). *Summary of the HIPAA privacy rules.* Retrieved from http://www.hhs.gov/ocr/privacy/hipaa/understanding/summary/

U.S. Department of Health and Human Services. (2013, February 11). *Construction of LMS Parameters for the Centers for Disease Control and Prevention 2000 Growth Charts,* by Katherine M. Flegal, Ph.D., Office of the Director, National Center for Health Statistics; and Tim J. Cole, Ph.D., MRC Centre of Epidemiology for Child Health, Institute of Child Health, University College London, UK. National Health Statistics Report (No. 63). Retrieved from http://www.cdc.gov/nchs/data/nhsr/nhsr063.pdf

U.S. Department of Health and Human Services, National Institutes of Health. (n.d.). *What health information is protected by the privacy rule?* Retrieved from http://privacyruleandresearch.nih.gov/pr_07.asp

U.S. Drug Enforcement Administration. (n.d.). Retrieved from www.dea.gov

U.S. Food and Drug Administration. (2013, April 1). *CFR - Code of Federal Regulations Title 21.* Retrieved from http://www.accessdata.fda.gov/scripts/cdrh/cfdocs/cfCFR/CFRSearch.cfm?fr=155.3